The Code Stroke Handbook

T0198121

The Code Stroke Handbook
Approach to the Acute Stroke Patient

ANDREW MICIELI, MD

Senior Neurology Resident, University of Toronto, Toronto, ON, Canada

RAED JOUNDI, MD, DPhil, FRCPC

Neurologist and Stroke Fellow, University of Calgary, Calgary, AB, Canada

HOUMAN KHOSRAVANI, MD, PhD, FRCPC

Assistant Professor, Division of Neurology, Department of Medicine, University of Toronto, Toronto, ON, Canada

Division of Neurology, Department of Medicine, Hurvitz Brain Sciences Program, and Regional Stroke Centre, Sunnybrook Health Sciences Centre, Neurology Quality and Innovation Lab (NQIL), Toronto, ON, Canada

JULIA HOPYAN, MBBS, FRACP, FRCPC

Assistant Professor, Division of Neurology, Department of Medicine, University of Toronto, Toronto, ON, Canada

Division of Neurology, Department of Medicine, Hurvitz Brain Sciences Program, and Regional Stroke Centre, Sunnybrook Health Sciences Centre, Toronto, ON, Canada

DAVID J. GLADSTONE, BSc, MD, PhD, FRCPC

Associate Professor, Division of Neurology, Department of Medicine, University of Toronto, Toronto, ON, Canada

Division of Neurology, Department of Medicine, Hurvitz Brain Sciences Program, and Regional Stroke Centre, Sunnybrook Health Sciences Centre, and Sunnybrook Research Institute, Toronto, ON, Canada

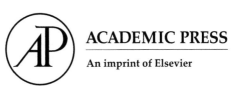

ACADEMIC PRESS

An imprint of Elsevier

ELSEVIER

Academic Press is an imprint of Elsevier
125 London Wall, London EC2Y 5AS, United Kingdom
525 B Street, Suite 1650, San Diego, CA 92101, United States
50 Hampshire Street, 5th Floor, Cambridge, MA 02139, United States
The Boulevard, Langford Lane, Kidlington, Oxford OX5 1GB, United Kingdom

Notices
Knowledge and best practice in this field are constantly changing. As new research and
experience broaden our understanding, changes in research methods, professional
practices, or medical treatment may become necessary.

Practitioners and researchers must always rely on their own experience and knowledge
in evaluating and using any information, methods, compounds, or experiments
described herein. In using such information or methods they should be mindful of their
own safety and the safety of others, including parties for whom they have a professional
responsibility.

To the fullest extent of the law, neither the Publisher nor the authors, contributors, or
editors, assume any liability for any injury and/or damage to persons or property as a
matter of products liability, negligence or otherwise, or from any use or operation of any
methods, products, instructions, or ideas contained in the material herein.

Library of Congress Cataloging-in-Publication Data
A catalog record for this book is available from the Library of Congress

British Library Cataloguing-in-Publication Data
A catalogue record for this book is available from the British Library

ISBN: 978-0-12-820522-8

For information on all Academic Press publications
visit our website at https://www.elsevier.com/books-and-journals

Last digit is the print number: 9   8   7   6   5

Publisher: Nikki Levy
Acquisitions Editor: Natalie Farra
Editorial Project Manager: Kristi Anderson
Production Project Manager: Omer Mukthar
Cover Designer: Mark Rogers
Cover Image: Andrew Micieli

Typeset by SPi Global, India

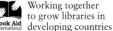

Working together
to grow libraries in
developing countries

www.elsevier.com • www.bookaid.org

Contents

4. Stroke Syndromes

5. Stroke Imaging: Noncontrast Head CT

6. Stroke Imaging: CT Angiography

7. Stroke Imaging: CT Perfusion

8. Acute Ischemic Stroke Treatment: Alteplase

Preface

A 65-year-old patient arrives at the Emergency Department with stroke symptoms that began 45 min ago. You are called STAT!

Acute stroke management has changed dramatically in recent years. Tremendous advances have been made in acute treatments, diagnostic neuroimaging, and organized systems of care, and are enabling better outcomes for patients. Stroke has evolved from a largely untreatable condition in the acute phase to a true medical emergency that is potentially treatable—and sometimes curable. The Code Stroke Emergency Response refers to a coordinated team-based approach to stroke patient care that requires rapid and accurate assessment, diagnosis, and treatment in an effort to save the brain and minimize permanent damage.

The Code Stroke Handbook contains the "essentials" of acute stroke to help clinicians provide best practice patient care

Designed to assist frontline physicians, nurses, paramedics, and medical learners at different levels of training, this book highlights clinical pearls and pitfalls, guideline recommendations, and other high-yield information not readily available in standard textbooks. It is filled with practical tips to prepare you for the next stroke emergency and reduce the anxiety you may feel when the Code Stroke pager rings.

❏ An easy-to-read, practical clinical resource spread over 12 chapters covering the basics of code stroke consultations—history taking, stroke mimics, neurological examination, acute stroke imaging (noncontrast CT/CT angiography/CT perfusion), and treatment (thrombolysis and endovascular therapy).

❏ Includes clinical pearls and pitfalls, neuroanatomy diagrams, and stroke syndromes, presented in an easily digestible format and book size that is convenient to carry around for quick reference when on-call at the hospital.

❏ Provides foundational knowledge for medical students and residents before starting their neurology, emergency medicine, or internal medicine rotations.

This book is dedicated to our patients with stroke, their families, and our colleagues, teachers, and mentors who have taught us so much.

We hope you enjoy this book.

Andrew Micieli
Raed Joundi
Houman Khosravani
Julia Hopyan
David J. Gladstone

Acknowledgments

Andrew Micieli has no academic acknowledgments. Dr. Joundi's stroke fellowship is funded by the Canadian Institutes of Health Research. Dr. Khosravani is supported by the Department of Medicine, Sunnybrook Health Sciences Centre; University of Toronto Centre for Quality Improvement and Patient Safety; and Thrombosis Canada. Dr. Hopyan is supported by the Department of Medicine, Sunnybrook Health Sciences Centre. Dr. Gladstone is supported by the Department of Medicine, Sunnybrook Health Sciences Centre; the Bastable-Potts Chair; the Tory family; and a Mid-Career Investigator Award from the Heart and Stroke Foundation of Canada.

CHAPTER 1

History taking

Beep…Beep…Beep
CODE STROKE in the Emergency Department,
Acute zone bed 10.

Welcome to the code stroke; let's get started.

The initial assessment of the code stroke patient involves identifying whether the clinical presentation is compatible with an acute stroke diagnosis or a stroke mimic. The first two chapters of this book will help answer this question. Like a good detective, you need to gather the important clues, ignore distractions and red herrings, and eliminate the other suspects—all in a timely manner. This chapter will provide you with a stepwise approach to:

❏ Taking an appropriate and focused history by gathering relevant clinical information from multiple sources.

❏ Identifying the common symptoms associated with (and not associated with) acute stroke.

Chapter 2 will discuss various stroke mimics and how to clinically differentiate them.

Early stroke symptom recognition is important to facilitate rapid transfer to a stroke center. Regional Emergency Medical Services (EMS) have protocols in place to identify and prioritize potential stroke cases, and try to minimize transportation time to the most appropriate stroke center. The mnemonic FAST, which stands for Face (sudden facial droop), Arm (sudden unilateral arm weakness), Speech (sudden speech difficulty), and Time to call EMS, is being used to promote public awareness. Most prehospital stroke screening tools involve some combination of these cardinal symptoms.

It has been estimated that nearly two million neurons die each minute that elapses during the evolution of an average acute ischemic stroke. Each hour without treatment the brain loses on average as many neurons as 3.6 years of normal aging. This is captured by a commonly used phrase "time is brain."

Ideal stroke treatment targets

❏ Door-to-needle time for intravenous tissue plasminogen activator (tPA): < 30 min
❏ Door-to-groin puncture time for endovascular therapy: < 60 min

Disability decreases with quicker treatment; therefore, aim for the fastest assessment for potential brain-saving or lifesaving treatment.

For the resident physcian or medical student on call, the first task is a simple one: write down the time you first received the code stroke page. There are many other time-related parameters that you may need to document throughout the code stroke, including time of patient arrival, time of the first CT scan slice, and time of tPA administration. This becomes important later when calculating *door-to-CT scan* time or *door-to-needle* time. After all, the quicker a stroke patient is treated, the more likely they are to have a functionally independent outcome.

Regional variations exist in terms of code stroke triage in the emergency department (ED). Depending on the hospital, the pager may notify you where the stroke patient is in the ED (or on the inpatient hospital ward), or you may need to call the number on the pager to confirm you received the page, ask the location of the stroke patient, and their estimated time of arrival if they are not already in the ED.

Sometimes the ED charge nurse will have some additional information for you. This prenotification clinical information can vary in terms of how detailed it is. Sometimes it is very detailed with a high pretest probability for stroke, such as:

We have a 76-year-old woman from home with a witnessed onset at 1500 hours of aphasia and right face, arm and leg weakness.

At other times, the clinical information is vague and undifferentiated, such as:

"85-year-old man with confusion." This could be a number of neurological or non neurological conditions (more on stroke mimics to come in Chapter 2).

Not all activated code strokes are from the ED. Inhospital strokes (i.e., a patient admitted to the ward) also occur, though with less frequency. Your approach to the patient should be the same. Often, the patient's medical comorbidities or recent surgery precludes the use of tPA.

Once the code stroke is activated, many different people are set in motion (even before the stroke resident/staff make their way to the patient). The first step is a rapid assessment and rushing the patient to the CT scanner as quickly as possible. In some hospitals, prior to the CT scan, the nurses will insert two cubital fossa IV lines, complete a 12-lead ECG, and draw urgent bloods that are sent stat for: CBC, electrolytes, creatinine, coagulation profile, random blood glucose level, troponin and type and screen. This blood work will help with treatment decisions and contraindications to tPA.

You have now made your way to the stroke patient in the ED. Like any acute situation in medicine, do not forget the basics: ABCs—**A**irway, **B**reathing, **C**irculation. Quickly eyeball the patient and check the vital signs from the monitors or from EMS or the triage nurse. Make sure that the patient is protecting their airway and there are no immediate life-threatening issues. Luckily, this is typically not the case, although some patients have a depressed level of consciousness either from a devastating intracranial event or another systemic issue. If the patient looks unstable, do not hesitate to request help from an ED physician, or rapid response/ICU.

Important initial questions to ask

Make every effort to speak directly to the paramedics, the patient, patient's family, and any eyewitness to obtain the most reliable medical history. There are 6 key questions to ask first, before we get a more detailed history and understand exactly what happened (specific symptoms and chronology):

1. Clarify the time the patient was "last seen normal" and the exact time of onset of symptoms, or the time the patient was found with symptoms.
2. What are the main neurological deficits? Did they improve or worsen en route?
3. Relevant past medical history and medications (do they have known atrial fibrillation? Are they taking anticoagulant medications? Do they have an allergy to contrast dye?).

4. Baseline functional status and occupation.
5. If arriving by EMS: vitals en route, EMS cardiac rhythm (normal sinus or atrial fibrillation or other?), blood glucose.
6. Did they bypass a closer hospital en route?

(1) The most important initial question to clarify with the patient, family, or witness is the stroke onset time and the patient's "last seen normal time," as it starts the clock on eligibility for acute treatment, i.e., thrombolytic therapy with tPA and/or endovascular therapy. Sometimes the exact time of onset is unknown/uncertain or difficult to obtain, but *try to really pin it down*. Use clock time (i.e., 23:00), rather than "2 h ago," or "30 min ago."

If the patient woke up with symptoms (i.e., a wake-up stroke), when were they last seen well? Did they get up in the middle of the night to use the washroom and were they normal then? If the patient woke up with symptoms in the morning without previous awakenings, we must use their last seen normal time which is typically when they went to bed. A common reason for ineligibility for tPA is arrival at the hospital too late, beyond the time window for treatment (although this is an evolving area of clinical research, and advanced imaging may enable the use of tPA outside the traditional time window).

(2) Now we need to clarify the neurological deficits.

Clinical features in favor of an acute arterial stroke diagnosis:

❏ Sudden onset of persistent focal neurological symptoms

❏ Symptoms compatible with a vascular territory (see Chapter 4—stroke syndromes).

What is a transient ischemic attack (TIA)?

Definition: a clinical syndrome characterized by the sudden onset of focal neurological symptoms that resolve within 24 h (although typically lasting minutes) AND no infarction is visualized on brain imaging.

The symptoms are transient as blood flow is temporarily blocked and then restored. Perfusion is dependent on many local and systemic factors (migration of clot, collateral circulation, cardiac output, blood pressure, etc.).

These patients are at risk of recurrent stroke—especially within the first week of symptom onset—and require timely assessment and management.

Clinical pearl: Given the increasing availability of MRI with diffusion weighted sequences, many clinical events previously thought to be TIAs are in fact small ischemic strokes.

Specifically, what are the neurological symptoms? Are they acute? Are they stable, fluctuating, worsening, or improving? Acute stroke is a dynamic condition and it is important to ask EMS if the symptoms have improved compared to their initial assessment.

Was there a loss of consciousness or evidence of seizure (rhythmic activity, bitten tongue, bruising, incontinence)? Focal deficits can occasionally follow a seizure (postictal) and are transient (called Todd's paresis). Are there associated fever or infectious symptoms, or other systemic symptoms such as palpitations, chest pain, or shortness of breath?

Time course and duration of symptoms is important. Migraine auras by definition last between 5 and 60 min in adults; however, typically they last 20–30 min. Seizures on average occur for 30 s–3 min. Syncope is brief, lasting seconds. More on stroke mimics in the next chapter.

Clinical pearls—We will review examples of neurological symptoms typically *not* associated with stroke

Recurrent/stereotyped episodes of aphasia

Aphasia is a cortical phenomenon and repeated ischemia to the same cortical area can be caused by TIAs if there is significant intracranial occlusive disease. However, one should also consider focal seizures (ictal aphasia). Another less likely etiology is migraine aura which may occur without headache.

Isolated dysphagia

When dysphagia is acute in onset, stroke should be considered, although isolated dysphagia is rare. Often, clarification of the history reveals a subacute or chronic presentation in which case the differential diagnosis is broad and includes neurological and non neurological etiologies.

Lower motor neuron ("peripheral") facial weakness (i.e., Bell's Palsy)

This pattern of weakness involves the forehead and is usually due to a lesion in the ipsilateral facial nerve (seventh cranial nerve). Rarely, a lesion in the brainstem facial nucleus or fascicle can also result in a lower motor neuron CN 7 palsy, but is almost always accompanied by a nuclear sixth nerve palsy or other symptoms in this scenario.

Isolated anisocoria

You cannot attribute isolated anisocoria to a stroke without associated ptosis to suggest a Horner's syndrome (associated with carotid artery dissection), or ptosis with some deficits in the rectus muscles innervated by the third cranial nerve to suggest a third nerve palsy (assuming the patient is not comatose).

(3) What is their past medical history? Do they have a previous history of stroke/TIA?

Vascular risk factors include:
- ❏ Previous TIA/stroke
- ❏ Atrial fibrillation
- ❏ Hypertension
- ❏ Diabetes
- ❏ Dyslipidemia
- ❏ Coronary artery disease or congestive heart failure
- ❏ Valvular heart disease
- ❏ Smoking
- ❏ Obstructive sleep apnea
- ❏ Alcohol abuse
- ❏ Other less common factors: migraine, oral contraceptive agents, hormone replacement therapy, antiphospholipid antibody syndrome, infection, cancer
- ❏ Rare genetic conditions such as (cerebral autosomal dominant arteriopathy with subcortical infarcts and leukoencephalopathy (CADASIL)) or Fabry disease.

Any recent surgery or invasive procedures? Recent gastrointestinal bleeding, genitourinary bleeding, or other adverse bleeding events? Any known kidney or liver disease or malignancy? Any recent myocardial infarction or recent TIAs/strokes? Any prior intracranial hemorrhage? History of seizures? Recent headaches, neck pain, whiplash or trauma? Known allergies to drugs or X-ray contrast dye?

(4) What is their baseline functional status? What is their occupation? What is their cognitive baseline, and what are their goals of care/DNR status?

(5) Were they hyper/hypotensive en route? Does the cardiac rhythm strip show an irregularly irregular rhythm or abnormalities relating to myocardial infarction (ST elevation)? Are they hypoglycemic?

Severe hypoglycemia or hyperglycemia can result in focal neurological signs and altered consciousness that can mimic stroke and blood glucose should always be checked on arrival at ED or obtained from EMS.

Look at the rhythm strip from EMS and telemetry monitor in ED as it may identify atrial fibrillation.

(6) Did EMS bypass a hospital en route to your stroke center? This is a practical question as it may be relevant to local hospital repatriation policies at some centers.

<u>The history is extremely important</u>. This cannot be stressed enough. You may not get all of it initially, but try to hit the high-yield questions before you move on to quickly examine the patient.

In summary, the most important questions are:
❏ Clarify the stroke onset time and/or last seen normal time
❏ What are the main new deficits
❏ Baseline functional status
❏ Is the patient on anticoagulation or have a past medical history of bleeding
❏ Vital signs and glucose

It is not possible to reliably predict an ischemic from a hemorrhagic stroke type based on history or examination alone, which is why patients are not recommended to take antiplatelets or anticoagulants at onset of symptoms before a CT head is done (approximately 15% of stroke events in North America are hemorrhagic). **Neuroimaging is necessary to differentiate ischemic from hemorrhagic stroke.**

Clinical clues for a hemorrhagic etiology include:
❏ Patient on anticoagulation
❏ Head trauma
❏ Progressive neurological deterioration

❏ Decreased level of alertness
❏ Thunderclap headache
❏ Nausea/vomiting
❏ Brain tumor
❏ Bleeding diathesis
❏ Vascular malformation/aneurysm

Improvement or recovery shortly after the onset of neurological deficit argues against a hemorrhagic etiology. Hemorrhagic TIA mimics exist, but are rare. However, remember that these clinical clues are not specific.

A word about…. Time is brain

As noted earlier, on average, approximately two million neurons are lost per minute in the setting of an acute stroke. This, however, is more variable depending on the patient's physiologic factors (e.g., hemodynamics, collateral blood supply) and can range from 35,000 up to 27 million neurons per minute. All of this means that when a code stroke is activated, a team has to assemble and carry out a series of defined tasks and execute them with precision. A series of interventions have been described in order to facilitate rapid registration, clinical assessment, neuroimaging, and decision-making with regard to acute stroke treatment.

It goes without saying that a cohesive team that is able to function well, communicate effectively, and rapidly assess and transition the patient in the emergency department from triage to the CT scanner is a key ingredient. Having an effective partnership with local EMS providers, and understanding the systems of care and patterns of referral are important. Some interventions that have been described to improve assessment times and door-to-needle and/or to groin puncture times and acute stroke management include the following:

- Engagement with EMS providers/systems of care
- Stroke center prenotification about the arrival of the patient, ideally with some personal health information
- Splitting up the tasks among the code stroke team members. Tasks to be split include: eliciting the history from EMS and family, examining the patient, looking up previous medical records in the electronic medical records system, checking previous and current blood work, and talking to family members to obtain a more detailed history and contraindications to thrombolytic therapy
- Rapid triaging of the patient with IV insertion, blood work draw, rapid CT order entry, and transfer of the patient directly to the CT scanner as quickly as possible
- Delivery of thrombolytic agent to the CT scanner with the ability to administer on the CT scanner table
- Availability of CT angiogram to assess for proximal occlusion and systems in place to proceed directly to the angiosuite or transfer the patient to an endovascular therapy-capable center
- Rapid neurologic assessment pre- and post-CT
- Rapid imaging protocols, optimized image transition from the scanner to the electronic medical system with appropriate advanced imaging, and rapid radiology interpretation.
- Patient disposition—transfer to appropriate monitored setting

Taken together, such interventions in the setting of teamwork can truly improve the workflow processes required to honor the phrase "time is brain."

As part of a process of continuous quality improvement, hospital-based stroke teams should rehearse their code stroke protocols, identify and correct local process or system issues that introduce delays to treatment, and monitor their local door-to-needle treatment times and other metrics in order to maximize efficiency. Regular education, case conferences, and feedback to team members about performance and patient outcomes are recommended.

In the context of the current COVID-19 pandemic caused by the SARS-CoV-2 virus, the ability to deliver timely and efficacious care must be balanced with the risk of infectious exposure to the clinical team. Therefore, we proposed modifications to routine hyperacute processes to account for COVID-19. Specific infection prevention and control recommendations were considered by adding clinical screening criteria. In addition, we recommended nuanced considerations for the healthcare team (using appropriate personal protective equipment), thereby modifying the conventional code stroke protocol in order to achieve a "protected" designation.

Summary

The history is an important part of the code stroke assessment. Based on the history gathered, you will have a low or high pretest probability for a stroke prior to the CT scan. Remember the six important questions to ask, specifically the time last seen normal, as it starts the clock on potential acute stroke therapy. Sometimes the onset of symptoms is vague, but try your best to clarify it. Vascular risk factors and a history of risk factors such as atrial fibrillation or nonadherence to antithrombotic therapy (ask when the last dose of anticoagulation was taken) are important information to gather.

Further reading

1. Boulanger JM, et al. Canadian stroke best practice recommendations for acute stroke management: prehospital, emergency department, and acute inpatient stroke care, 6th edition, update 2018. *Int J Stroke*. 2018;13(9):949–984.
2. Caplan L. *Caplan's Stroke. A Clinical Approach*. 4th ed. Boston: Elsevier Canada; 2009.
3. Caplan LR, Biller J, Leary M, et al. *Primer on Cerebrovascular Diseases*. Academic Press; 2017.
4. Saver JL. Time is brain–quantified. *Stroke*. 2006;37(1):263–266.
5. Desai SM, Rocha M, Jovin TG, Jadhav AP. High variability in neuronal loss. *Stroke*. 2019;50:34–37.
6. Meretoja A, Strbian D, Mustanoja S, Tatlisumak T, Lindsberg PJ, Kaste M. Reducing in-hospital delay to 20 minutes in stroke thrombolysis. *Neurology*. 2012;79:306–313.
7. Kamal N, Benavente O, Boyle K, et al. Good is not good enough: The benchmark stroke door-to-needle time should be 30 minutes. *Can J Neurol Sci*. 2014;41:694–696.
8. Hill MD, Coutts SB. Alteplase in acute ischaemic stroke: the need for speed. *Lancet*. 2014;384:1904–1906.
9. Khosravani H, et al. Protected Code Stroke: Hyperacute Stroke Management During the Coronavirus Disease 2019 (COVID-19) Pandemic. *Stroke*. 2020:STROKEAHA120029838. https://doi.org/10.1161/STROKEAHA.120.029838.

CHAPTER 2

Stroke mimics

This chapter will provide you with a broad differential diagnosis for acute stroke. We discuss clinical clues to identify the most common stroke mimics with case examples. Specifically, we will review how to differentiate a migraine, seizure, or psychogenic presentation from stroke. In addition, we will review important concepts which include differentiating peripheral from central vertigo, causes of a decreased level of consciousness in stroke, and recognition of stroke-related visual symptoms.

A good start is to ask yourself, "is this *likely or unlikely to be an acute stroke*?" and keep in mind the list below of potential stroke mimics.

- ❏ **Migraine with aura or migraine variants**
- ❏ **Seizure – ictal or post-ictal (e.g. Todd's paralysis)**
- ❏ **Psychogenic symptoms**
- ❏ **Presyncope or syncope**
- ❏ **Acute medical delirium**
- ❏ **Acute exacerbation (or unmasking) of old stroke symptoms/deficits**

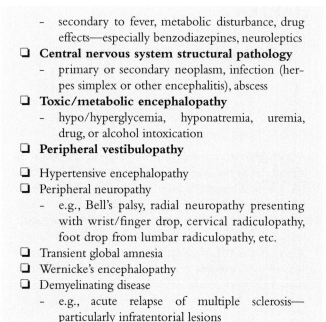

- secondary to fever, metabolic disturbance, drug effects—especially benzodiazepines, neuroleptics
❏ **Central nervous system structural pathology**
  - primary or secondary neoplasm, infection (herpes simplex or other encephalitis), abscess
❏ **Toxic/metabolic encephalopathy**
  - hypo/hyperglycemia, hyponatremia, uremia, drug, or alcohol intoxication
❏ **Peripheral vestibulopathy**

❏ Hypertensive encephalopathy
❏ Peripheral neuropathy
  - e.g., Bell's palsy, radial neuropathy presenting with wrist/finger drop, cervical radiculopathy, foot drop from lumbar radiculopathy, etc.
❏ Transient global amnesia
❏ Wernicke's encephalopathy
❏ Demyelinating disease
  - e.g., acute relapse of multiple sclerosis—particularly infratentorial lesions

The list of stroke mimics is very broad, and includes rare diagnoses not mentioned in the above table. Keep the bolded (most common) possibilities in mind when assessing the patient. Approximately 10%–20% of code strokes are stroke mimics. Prehospital screening criteria are designed to enhance sensitivity, rather than specificity, so as not to miss patients with a potentially treatable acute stroke. Although the risk of a tPA-related intracerebral hemorrhage in most stroke mimics is reported to be very low (approximately 0.5% from pooled analyses), every attempt should be made to achieve an accurate diagnosis before treatment.

Below we will discuss some clues to help you differentiate a stroke from the common mimics based on symptomatology. Careful history taking is essential.

1 What are clinical clues to differentiate seizure or migraine aura from stroke/TIA?

❏ Stroke symptoms are typically negative symptoms. This indicates a *loss of function*, such as weakness, anesthesia or decreased sensation, or loss of vision. In contrast, positive symptoms indicate overactivity of central nervous system neurons, and are typical of seizures (ictal phase) and migraine auras. Positive symptoms include bright or flashing lights/shapes/objects, scintillating scotomas (migraine visual auras are often crescentic with zigzag or jagged edges or shimmering borders, and may expand or move in the visual field before disappearing), paresthesias (a pins and needles tingling sensation), and rhythmic clonic movements.

❏ Stroke symptoms are typically sudden in onset, particularly embolic stroke events (in some cases, small vessel lacunar syndromes may stutter and progress in a stepwise or gradual fashion). Seizures or migraines typically have a *march* or spread of symptoms from one body part to another over time. The patient with a migraine sensory aura may say: "The fingers of my left hand started tingling, and the tingling spread up my left arm and then into the left side of my cheek, lips, and tongue over a few minutes." A postictal motor deficit (i.e., cortical suppression) may follow an unwitnessed focal onset seizure. This can last for hours, mimicking a stroke.

Case presentation

A code stroke is activated for a 64-year-old gentleman brought in by EMS with "left-sided weakness." His past medical history is significant for a right middle cerebral artery infarct 6 months ago. He is on aspirin, atorvastatin, and perindopril and is compliant with his medications.

His neuroimaging with a noncontrast head CT, CT angiogram, and CT perfusion shows his old right cerebral cortical infarct but does not reveal new acute ischemic changes, intracranial vessel occlusion, or perfusion abnormality. His CT angiogram also does not show any significant carotid or vertebrobasilar artery stenosis.

You assess the patient and after clarifying the history further, you correctly identify that he first noticed his left arm started to "shake," followed by his left leg for about 30 s. After cessation of these abnormal movements, his left arm/leg was weak at which point his family noticed the weakness and called EMS.

Summary: *This patient had a focal motor seizure with preserved awareness followed by a post-ictal Todd's Paralysis. The focal seizure was secondary to his chronic right cerebral infarct.*

At times it can be more difficult to identify what came first. Patients can have seizures at the onset of an acute stroke or afterward, although this is uncommon. Neuroimaging, particularly CT angiography, can be very helpful in such cases.

Clinical pearl: There are exceptions to the rule. Positive symptoms can be seen in acute stroke such as hemichorea, hemiballismus, or hemidystonia in basal ganglia infarctions, although this is rare. Rhythmic tonic–clonic movements can occasionally be seen in some brainstem infarcts and limb shaking TIAs which we will discuss next. Speech arrest can be seen in focal seizures.

2 Limb shaking TIA

Limb shaking TIAs are an uncommon form of TIA, but a phenomenon that we should recognize. The mechanism is typically hemodynamic in the setting of severe carotid disease. Correct recognition is important as treatment involves carotid revascularization. There are clinical cues that may help differentiate a vascular etiology from a focal seizure; however, in clinical practice, it is difficult. These include:

❏ Presence of precipitating maneuvers causing cerebral hypoperfusion such as getting up from a bed or chair, hyperextending the neck, hyperventilation, or resolution of symptoms after sitting or lying down.

❏ Absence of tongue biting or Jacksonian march.

❏ EEG does not show epileptiform activity (however this could also be the case for focal seizures in the interictal period).

❏ Anticonvulsant medications are not effective.

Another cause of fluctuating hemiparesis is the <u>capsular warning syndrome, which typically presents with relapsing and remitting hemiparesis</u>.

Capsular warning syndrome ("stuttering lacune")

This is a specific stroke syndrome presenting with recurrent, stereotyped lacunar TIAs. The symptomatology is usually recurrent episodes of hemiparesis due to internal capsule ischemia. It is attributed to local ischemia from an occluded/occluding single small penetrating vessel. This syndrome is associated with a high risk of developing a completed stroke with permanent deficits.

This symptomatology could be confused with that of nonvascular etiology, such as a focal motor seizure.

3 Migraine

Migraine is very common in the general population, and can begin at any age. Migraine auras can occur with or without a headache. If headache is present, ask about head pain quality (throbbing, pulsating), associated photophobia, phonophobia, nausea, vomiting, and aggravation with activity. In acephalgic migraine, aura occurs without a headache, further confusing the picture.

Below is a table highlighting the different migraine types that may mimic a stroke or TIA. Remember that in the acute stroke setting, migraine and seizure are best diagnosed after stroke has been ruled out (i.e., diagnosis of exclusion).

Migraine mimics

Migraine with aura

❏ An aura consists of visual, sensory, or speech/language symptoms, each fully reversible (without motor symptoms). An aura spreads gradually over 5 min and typically lasts 5–60 min. The aura is followed (within 60 min) by a headache.

❏ Transient sensory symptoms, aphasia or negative symptoms associated with migraine may be clinically challenging to diagnosis. The sensory aura can be paresthesias or numbness, typically involving face and hand. Visual auras mostly comprise positive symptoms (scintillating scotoma, fortification spectra, kaleidoscopic vision), but negative symptoms can also occur (often following a positive visual phenomenon), including loss of vision such as a hemifield deficit or visual scotoma. It can be helpful to show patients pictures of the different types of visual auras to see if any resemble the patient's aura (simply google "migraine visual aura").

❑ In some patients, an aura is not followed by a migraine, which is seen in *typical aura without headache* (i.e., acephalgic migraine).

Migraine with brainstem aura

❑ Previously known as basilar artery migraine; basilar migraine; basilar-type migraine.

❑ In addition to the typical aura discussed above, they also have *at least* two brainstem symptoms such as dysarthria, vertigo, tinnitus, hypacusis, diplopia, ataxia, or decreased level of consciousness. Each individual aura symptom lasts between 5 and 60 min. Onset is more common in pediatrics, but there are late-onset cases.

Hemiplegic migraine

❑ Both a typical aura and *fully reversible objective motor weakness* must be present (do not need complete hemiplegia for diagnosis). The motor weakness typically lasts <72 h.

❑ The attacks can have sequelae that last for hours, days, weeks, and rarely permanent deficits. There are three well-described genotypes of familial hemiplegia migraine (autosomal dominant transmission). These patients are younger than the typical stroke patient, with their first episodes usually starting before 20 years of age.

❑ Hemiplegic migraine is a <u>diagnosis of exclusion</u>. It is very rare with a prevalence of 0.01%.

HaNDL = Headache and neurologic deficits with cerebrospinal fluid lymphocytosis

❑ It is a rare, self-limited, benign entity generally lasting 15–120 min. Like hemiplegic migraine, it is a diagnosis of exclusion.

❑ The headache is moderate-severe, often associated with nausea and vomiting. The most frequent neurologic symptoms associated with HaNDL are hemiparesis, hemisensory disturbances, and aphasia, and visual symptoms are less common.

❑ CSF must have > 15 WBC.

Thunderclap headache is a very sudden onset, severe headache, often described as the "worst headache of my life." By definition, the pain reaches its maximum intensity in < 1 min (often within a few seconds). It has a broad differential diagnosis, of which the most worrisome is bleeding into the subarachnoid space (subarachnoid hemorrhage), from a ruptured intracranial aneurysm. Other etiologies, and relevant to stroke, include reversible cerebral vasoconstriction syndrome (RCVS), cerebral venous thrombosis, and arterial dissection. The recommended imaging test is an immediate noncontrast head CT to look for hemorrhage, followed by a contrast-enhanced CT angiogram to look for aneurysm, vascular malformation, and other pathology.

4 Clinical cues to help differentiate a peripheral from a central cause of vertigo

Firstly, dizziness is a nonspecific and imprecise term that can mean different things to different patients. Try to clarify what patients mean when they say they are dizzy or vertiginous. Are their symptoms consistent with vertigo, lightheadedness, disequilibrium, or oscillopsia? **Vertigo** is an illusion of movement of self or the environment, often rotatory, and persists with eyes closed (can be central or peripheral in etiology). In contrast, patients with presyncope describe a feeling faint or lightheaded as if they are going to pass out. **Dysequilibrium** is a sensation of imbalance when standing or walking (it is typically nonspecific with a large differential diagnosis). **Oscillopsia** is an illusory movement (usually rhythmic) of the environment which disappears with eyes closed. This can be due to nystagmus, or an impaired vestibulo–ocular reflex which occurs when the head is moving.

Try to characterize the course, duration, associated symptoms, or provoking factors of the vertigo.

❏ Is it constant or episodic?

❏ Are there provoking factors (such as specific head movements or anxiety) or is it spontaneous?

❏ Is it positional (lying down, sitting up, changing position in bed)? Ask patients if the dizziness is precipitated by head turning to the right or left, or with neck extension, or is orthostatic (when arising from bed or chair).

❏ Does it occur with eyes open or closed?

❏ Are there any associated neurological symptoms such as diplopia, dysarthria, clumsiness/incoordination of limbs, focal weakness, or sensory symptoms, impairment in walking or balance? Hiccups can be a clue to brainstem ischemia (e.g., lateral medullary stroke).

❏ Is there nausea or vomiting?

❏ Have they experienced previous episodes?

❏ Was there a preceding upper respiratory illness?

❏ Did they recently start a new medication?

There are many different etiologies for peripheral vertigo such as benign paroxysmal positional vertigo (BPPV), recurrent vestibulopathy, vestibular neuronitis, Meniere's disease, trauma (such as a temporal bone fracture), and medication toxicity (e.g., gentamicin ear drops).

Below is a clinical guide to help differentiate peripheral from central vertigo. These are not absolute and patients often do not fit nicely into one of the categories. Neuroimaging is helpful *and often needed*.

	Factors favoring peripheral vertigo	Factors favoring central vertigo
Onset	Acute/sudden	Acute/sudden
Duration	Intermittent (seconds to hours)	Constant

(Continued)

	Factors favoring peripheral vertigo	Factors favoring central vertigo
Provoking factors	Head movement/ positional	Rare
Associated neurological symptoms	Absent	Usually (unless small cerebellar infarct). Do not forget to check the patient's gait and balance. A gait ataxia suggests a cerebellar, brainstem, or thalamic lesion
Associated auditory symptoms	Decreased hearing, tinnitus, ear fullness	Absent (exception is an anterior inferior cerebellar artery (AICA) stroke with labyrinthine artery involvement)
Nausea/ vomiting	Often present and moderate-to-severe	If present, often mild-to-moderate severity
Preceding event	Upper respiratory illness, trauma	None
Postural and gait instability	Often less severely affected	More severely affected. May fall toward the side of the lesion
Past medical history	May have a history of previous vertigo attacks, ear infection, or migraine	May have vascular risk factors
Medications	Anticonvulsants, antibiotics (cisplatin and aminoglycosides)	None

	Factors favoring peripheral vertigo	Factors favoring central vertigo
Nystagmus	Typically mixed horizontal-torsional (fast phase *away* from the side of the lesion)	May have any trajectory (i.e., purely vertical, torsional, horizontal) or a mixed waveform. It can reverse direction when looking right, then left (periodic alternating nystagmus) Isolated vertical nystagmus is rarely ever peripheral.
	The predominant direction of nystagmus remains the same in all directions of gaze	
	Visual fixation may suppress nystagmus	<u>Downbeat nystagmus</u> localizes to either the dorsal medulla or cerebellar flocculus (or its projections). <u>Upbeat nystagmus</u> localizes to the cerebellum or brainstem
		It is not suppressed by vision
		The absence of these features does not rule out a central cause of vertigo

5 Stroke and decreased level of consciousness

Oftentimes, a code stroke is activated for a patient with an altered level of consciousness (LOC). If there are no focal neurological signs, physicians often consider other neurological conditions (seizure, encephalopathy, or central nervous system infection) or systemic/metabolic abnormalities.

However, strokes can present with decreased LOC, altered mental status, or confusion, and can be life threatening.

For a stroke to cause decreased LOC, it must localize to either the:

  (i) Reticular activating system in the brainstem—there should be accompanying brainstem clinical signs such as oculomotor deficits, dysarthria, facial, or limb weakness.
 (ii) Unilateral or bilateral thalamus
(iii) Bilateral hemispheres (e.g., shower of multiple emboli)—in which case other focal deficits may or may not be noted.

Clinical pearl: Sudden unconsciousness can be a presenting symptom of basilar artery occlusion, which can be rapidly ruled in or ruled out by a CT angiogram. If basilar occlusion is suspected, it should be ruled out immediately.

Large right MCA infarcts may have inattention, eye closure (apraxia of eyelid opening), and the appearance of drowsiness.

A large unilateral infarct or hemorrhage with midline shift, or malignant cerebral edema also leads to decreased LOC.

Case presentation

You are on call overnight and are paged by the ED physician for an 84-year-old woman with an acute drop in her level of consciousness. She has a past medical history of hypertension, dyslipidemia, and hypothyroidism. In the ED they noticed intermittent, transient "generalized tremulousness" prior to intubation for her low level of consciousness. A noncontrast head CT was completed in the ED and is reported as normal.

On your assessment she opens her eyes to painful stimuli and withdraws to pain on the right side. She has a right internuclear ophthalmoplegia (INO), pinpoint pupils, intermittent and tran-

sient jerking/shivering movements, and plantar reflexes are extensor bilaterally.

You order a stat CT angiogram of the head and neck vessels confirming the diagnosis of a mid-basilar artery occlusion. You urgently assess for tPA and call the neuro-interventionalist for endovascular thrombectomy.

<u>Summary:</u> *Basilar artery occlusions can present in many ways, and may result in a sudden onset loss of consciousness or a gradually progressive decrease in consciousness as a result of interruption of the reticular activating system in the brainstem. A clinical pearl is the look for the presence of abnormal eye findings or other brainstem signs, and also abnormal movements that can be seen in this syndrome, which include jerking, tremor, twitching, or shivering. These movements may be misdiagnosed as seizures. An urgent CT and CT angiogram of the head and neck is indicated to assess the posterior circulation.*

We will review imaging of basilar occlusions in the neuroimaging chapters, and Chapter 10 will specifically review basilar artery occlusions.

6 Stroke and visual symptoms

Stroke patients often have visual symptoms and early recognition is important for acute treatment and prevention of further events. What visual symptoms are related to a vascular event and what urgent neuroimaging is required? The first question to determine is:

6.1 Are the visual symptoms monocular or binocular?

(i) Monocular vision loss

Acute monocular vision loss may be transient or permanent. Either way, monocular symptoms imply a disorder anterior to the optic chiasm (i.e., the optic nerve or the eye). A clinical pearl is often patients with binocular vision loss such as a homonymous hemianopia, localize the problem to the eye with the temporal visual field defect since the temporal visual field is larger than the nasal field. Check the visual fields in each eye separately.

Sudden painless vision loss in one eye suggests vascular etiologies such as a <u>central retinal artery occlusion (CRAO)</u> or a <u>branch retinal artery occlusion (BRAO)</u>. The differential diagnosis also includes entities such as ischemic optic neuropathy, central retinal vein occlusion, retinal detachment, or vitreous hemorrhage, indicating the importance of obtaining an urgent ophthalmology consultation in such cases.

❏ Central retinal artery occlusion presents with painless, often severe vision loss in one eye. This may be the only symptom of an embolic stroke and if this diagnosis is confirmed with a dilated fundus examination, tPA may be considered. Branch retinal artery occlusion will usually cause an altitudinal visual field defect (i.e., vision loss in the superior or inferior half of the eye) rather than the diffuse loss seen with a CRAO. This is because the embolus lodges more distally in the retinal circulation.

❏ <u>Giant cell arteritis (GCA)</u> should be considered in your differential diagnosis of any patient over 50 years of age with sudden painless monocular vision loss. Ischemic optic neuropathy is the most common cause of vision loss in GCA, but CRAO is also possible. When GCA causes a CRAO, there is no embolus visible in the retinal circulation. Patients with vision loss from GCA may or may not have the other systemic symptoms characteristic of the disease (i.e., temporal headache, jaw claudication, scalp tenderness, or myalgias), and a CBC, ESR, and CRP should be obtained when the diagnosis is suspected. The superficial temporal arteries should be examined and should be soft, pulsatile, and non-tender (normal). If they are hard, distended, non-pulsatile, and tender to palpation, it is suspicious for giant cell arteritis.

Transient monocular vision loss also has a large differential diagnosis that includes ocular surface disease (i.e., dry eyes), intermittent angle closure, impending retinal vein occlusion, or transient ischemia to the retina or optic nerve. A retinal TIA has characteristic features such as sudden onset, duration of a few minutes, and often patients describe a dark curtain being pulled down or up over the affected eye, or "lamp shade" that lifts up after resolution. The ocular fundus will be normal in patients with a retinal TIA. In a patient with a suspected retinal TIA, a stroke workup is indicated since these patients are at risk for ischemic stroke. A CT angiogram (starting at the aortic arch), echocardiogram, and Holter monitoring is indicated to identify a treatable thromboembolic source from the heart, aortic arch, or carotid artery.

❏ Giant cell arteritis should be considered in patients with transient monocular vision loss. A large proportion of patients with permanent vision loss from GCA describe preceding episodes of transient vision loss before they lose vision.

(ii) Binocular vision loss
Binocular vision loss may also be transient or permanent. When the retrochiasmal visual structures are involved, a homonymous hemianopia or quadrantanopia visual field defect is produced. Homonymous means that the vision loss is similar in both eyes. A complete homonymous hemianopia localizes to the contralateral retrochiasmal

visual pathway (optic tract, optic radiations, or occipital lobe). Visual acuity is preserved in all homonymous visual field defects unless the process is bilateral or there is additional pathology in the anterior visual pathways. As an example, a complete MCA territory stroke (from a proximal MCA occlusion) will result in a contralateral homonymous hemianopia, as will a complete posterior cerebral artery (PCA) territory stroke. A superior MCA trunk infarct (with involvement of the parietal lobe) can result in an inferior quadrantanopia. In contrast, an inferior MCA trunk infarct (with involvement of the temporal lobe) can result in a superior quadrantanopia.

❏ A rare cause of bilateral sudden vision loss is posterior ischemic optic neuropathy (PION). This is typically seen in the context of giant cell arteritis or in the perioperative setting when there is significant hypotension or anemia. The ocular examination is normal in the acute setting in PION.

6.2 Diplopia

Binocular diplopia results from a misalignment of the eyes (usually due to a nerve or muscle palsy) and resolves when either eye is occluded. It may be the presenting symptom of a brainstem ischemic stroke. When this is the case, it is due to vertebrobasilar ischemia/infarction from involvement of the oculomotor nuclei, nerves, or supra/internuclear pathways. Typically, there are other brainstem symptoms and double vision is not usually seen in isolation. There is also a large differential diagnosis for diplopia, and stroke is the cause in a small proportion of patients. An ophthalmology or neuro–ophthalmology consultation should be considered if the etiology is unclear.

7 What clues on history suggest a psychogenic disorder?

A psychogenic or "functional" disorder implies that the symptoms arise from abnormal nervous system functioning in the absence of structural pathology. Examples include anxiety, panic attack, somatic symptom disorder, illness anxiety disorder (hypochondriasis), conversion disorder, and factitious disorder (consult the DSM for diagnostic criteria). Functional weakness, sensory symptoms, dizziness, or visual symptoms can be challenging to sort out clinically, as they can present with acute/sudden onset deficits mimicking a stroke. Up to 30% of all stroke mimics may be accounted for by a functional disorder. These patients are typically younger than the average stroke patient. Patients with organic dysfunction can also have a level of functional overlay making interpretation of clinical findings even more difficult. Below are some clinical clues but none are absolute and the diagnosis can be difficult for even the most seasoned clinicians, especially during an initial emergency assessment. However, remember that a functional disorder remains a diagnosis of exclusion in the acute setting. A more detailed history taking and examination, and repeated assessments, are often necessary.

Clinical clues to help distinguish a functional disorder

❏ Symptoms may be preceded by an emotional trigger or anxiety-provoking situation.
❏ Minute-to-minute fluctuations in weakness.

❏ Nonneuroanatomical pattern of motor or sensory deficits.

❏ Stuttering speech.

❏ Selective mutism (can comprehend and write perfectly perfectly, in contrast to patients who are truly aphasic, in which impairment in reading and writing is usually present in addition to speech impairment).

❏ Past history of trauma (physical or psychological), psychiatric diagnosis, or functional disorder.

We are now ready to move onto Chapter 3, the code stroke physical examination, but before we do so, let us go through a case.

Case presentation

A 76-year-old female from home presented to the ED with acute confusion. She has a past medical history of hypertension. When assessed by the emergency room physician she is speaking non-sense, and becomes very agitated when asked questions or when asked to perform specific tasks. A noncontrast head CT completed in the ED is normal. She is admitted to the internal medicine inpatient ward for a delirium workup. An MRI completed a few days later as part of the workup reveals a small left middle cerebral artery (MCA) acute infarct (inferior trunk of the MCA).

Case highlights: This specific MCA localization can be mistaken for hyperactive delirium. The inferior trunk of MCA supplies the lateral surface of the temporal lobe and the inferior parietal lobe. This patient had Wernicke's aphasia (see Chapter 3 for a bedside examination of aphasia) and had difficulty understanding questions or commands. These patients may not have accompanying motor or sensory symptoms (the primary motor and sensory cortices are not affected), making the diagnosis difficult. An important bedside exam maneuver is to test language function (to identify paraphasic errors or other signs of aphasia), and to check visual fields, as you may pick up a contralateral superior quadrantanopia, although this could be challenging if there is a language disturbance.

Summary

We reviewed several stroke mimics to be aware and think of during a code stroke, the most common ones being migraine, seizure, metabolic encephalopathy, and psychogenic. Keep an open mind and seek to document the pertinent positives and negatives to narrow down your differential diagnosis. At times you may need to rely on neuroimaging, which we will review shortly.

Further reading

1. Abdelnour LH, El-Nagi F. Functional neurological disorder presenting as stroke: a narrative review. *J Psychol Abnorm*. 2017;6:1.
2. Boulanger JM, et al. Canadian stroke best practice recommendations for acute stroke management: prehospital, emergency department, and acute inpatient stroke care, 6th edition, update 2018. *Int J Stroke*. 2018;13(9):949–984.
3. Caplan L. *Caplan's Stroke. A Clinical Approach*. 4th ed. Boston: Elsevier Canada; 2009.
4. Caplan LR, Biller J, Leary M, et al. *Primer on Cerebrovascular Diseases*. Academic Press; 2017.
5. https://www.uptodate.com/contents/jerk-nystagmus.
6. Liberman A, Prabhakaran S. Stroke Chameleons and stroke mimics in the emergency department. *Curr Neurol Neurosci Rep*. 2017;17(2):15.
7. Persoon S, Kappelle LJ, Klijn CJ. Limb-shaking transient ischaemic attacks in patients with internal carotid artery occlusion: a case-control study. *Brain*. 2010;133(3):915.

CHAPTER 3

NIH stroke scale and neurological examination

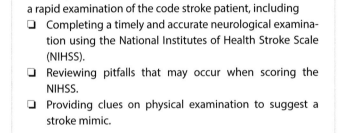

This chapter will provide you with an approach to conducting a rapid examination of the code stroke patient, including

❏ Completing a timely and accurate neurological examination using the National Institutes of Health Stroke Scale (NIHSS).

❏ Reviewing pitfalls that may occur when scoring the NIHSS.

❏ Providing clues on physical examination to suggest a stroke mimic.

Remember. This is not the full formal neurological examination we are accustomed to completing in a clinic or on the inpatient ward. Rather, this is a brief practical (on-the-fly, done-in-the-elevator) screening examination to assist with the rapid decision-making.

Parts of the standard neurological examination that are *not* included in the NIHSS score include:

❏ Cognitive assessment

❏ Visual acuity

❏ Pupils and Horner's syndrome

❏ Vertical eye movements and nystagmus

❏ Cranial nerves 8–12

❏ Muscle tone

❏ Formal power (muscle resistance) testing
❏ Distal limb weakness (e.g. hand/finger weakness)
❏ Reflexes
❏ Sensation to vibration, proprioception, and cortical sensation
❏ Romberg
❏ Gait assessment

After the action of the code stroke has settled, a more detailed neurological examination, including the above-mentioned sections can be completed and documented.

In the ideal situation, the full NIHSS is completed before the patient goes into the CT scanner. Practically, this is not always feasible, as it is the highest priority to get the patient to the scanner as soon as possible. Elements of the NIHSS are often performed while the patient is being transported to the scanner, or while the patient is being prepared to enter the scanner.

A few tips when performing the NIHSS under time pressure
❏ Weakness, language, and gaze deviation are likely the highest yield elements of the examination when assessing the likelihood of stroke and localization.
❏ Always include elements that are most relevant to the patient's presenting complaint/symptoms. For example, if the patient presents with visual impairment and sensory loss (posterior cerebral artery territory), you would miss the localization by focusing only on the motor or language assessment.
❏ Some parts of the examination can be done simply through inspection (level of consciousness, gaze preference, facial droop).
❏ The full NIHSS can be completed once the patent is out of the CT scanner, and supplemented with additional examination elements as needed.

❏ Lastly, introduce yourself to the team (RNs and others) and work with and around them to begin the process of examination as other assessments (i.e., application of hospital ID, bloodwork) are taking place.

Let us go through each section of the NIHSS. This scoring system is a reliable and valid clinical and research tool to measure the presence/absence and severity of neurological impairments. It is a 15 item scale, with total score ranging from 0 to 42 points (higher score indicates more severe deficits), which correlates with stroke size and can predict long-term outcomes after stroke (Figs. 3.1 and 3.2). However, an important concept to remember is that the number itself does not always equate to the level of disability, and disability needs to be considered on an individual basis depending on the type of deficits and specific characteristics of the patient (impact on work, hobbies, driving). For example, homonymous hemianopia results in difficulty reading and an inability to drive, neglect can be very disabling, and distal hand weakness (especially of the dominant hand) in a concert pianist can rob a person of their livelihood. Furthermore, while aphasia may only give a few points on the NIHSS, it can be a devastating deficit.

The NIHSS scoring system is weighted more heavily for dominant (left) hemisphere strokes since they can score more points for aphasia. It also underestimates (or can miss) posterior circulation stroke deficits.

A couple of pointers before we start:
❏ Do not go back and change scores
❏ Be as objective as possible
❏ Try to not coach the patient

NIHSS training (video tutorials) and certification modules are available online and are highly recommended for clinicians interested in acute stroke patient assessment

Here is a general guide on how to categorize the stroke severity using the NIHSS:

NIHSS score	Stroke severity	Brain tissue at risk of infarction
0–5	Mild	
6–10	Moderate	
11–20	Severe	
>20	Very severe	

Fig. 3.1   How to categorize stroke severity using the NIHSS.

1 National Institutes of Health Stroke Scale

(A)

1a. Level of consciousness	
0	Alert; keenly responsive
1	Not alert; but arousable by minor stimulation to obey, answer, or respond
2	Not alert; requires repeated stimulation to attend, or is obtunded and requires strong or painful stimulation to make movements (not stereotyped)
3	Responds only with reflex motor or autonomic effects or totally unresponsive, flaccid, and areflexic

The investigator should choose a response even in patients with endotracheal tubes, language barrier, orotracheal trauma/bandages, etc. A score of 3 is only given if the patient fails to respond (other than reflexive posturing) after noxious stimulation.

1b. LOC questions Ask the patient: "What month is it? How old are you?"	
0	Answers both correctly
1	Answers one correctly
2	Answers neither correctly

Score only the initial answer (there is no credit for being close). Patients unable to speak due to intubation, orotracheal trauma, severe dysarthria, language barrier, etc., are scored 1. Aphasic and stuporous patients are scored 2.

Fig. 3.2   (A) National Institute of Health Stroke Scale cards.

1c. LOC commands Command the patient to: "Open and close your eyes. Grip and release your hand"	
0	Performs both correctly
1	Performs one correctly
2	Performs neither correctly

Make sure the patient is asked to use the unaffected nonparetic hand. Substitute another command if the hands cannot be used. Score only the first attempt. Patients too weak to complete the command can be scored if they have made an unequivocal attempt to follow the command. If the patient is unresponsive, the task should be demonstrated.

2. Best gaze Establish eye contact and ask the patient to: "Follow my finger"	
0	Normal
1	Partial gaze palsy
2	Forced deviation or total gaze paresis

Appropriate for aphasic patients. Forced deviation or total gaze paresis is not overcome by the oculocephalic maneuver. Score voluntary or reflexive, horizontal eye movements (do not do the caloric test). Test patients with ocular trauma, bandages, preexisting blindness, etc., for reflexive movement and a choice is made by the investigator. Patients with a conjugate deviation of the eyes (overcome by voluntary or reflexive activity) and those with isolated peripheral nerve paresis (CN III, IV, or VI) are scored 1.

Fig. 3.2, cont'd

(Continued)

3. Visual fields **Use confrontation, finger counting, or visual threat.** **Confront upper/lower quadrants of visual field**	
0	No visual loss
1	Partial hemianopsia
2	Complete hemianopia
3	Bilateral hemianopsia

Test patients with unilateral blindness or enucleation in the remaining eye. Patients with clear-cut asymmetry, including quadrantanopia, are scored 1. Blind patients are scored 3.
Test again using double simultaneous stimulation. Score 1 for extinction and record under item 11.

4. Facial palsy **By words or pantomime, encourage the patient to:** **"Show me your teeth. Raise your eyebrows. Close** **your eyes"**	
0	Normal symmetrical movement
1	Minor paralysis (flattened nasolabial fold, asymmetry on smiling)
2	Partial paralysis (lower face)
3	Complete paralysis

If possible, remove facial bandages, orotracheal tube, tape, etc., before testing. In poorly responsive patients, score symmetry of grimace in response to noxious stimuli.

Fig. 3.2, cont'd

5. Arm motor
Alternately position patient's arms. Extend each arm with palms down (90 degrees if sitting, 45 degrees if supine)

0	No drift
1	Drift
2	Some effort vs gravity (arm drifts down to the bed)
3	No effort vs gravity
4	No movement
UN	Amputation or joint fusion

Test each arm in turn (nonparetic arm first). Drift is scored if arm falls before 10 s. Score untestable (UN) only for patients with amputations or joint fusions of the shoulder.

6. Leg motor
Alternately position patient's legs. Extend each leg (30 degrees, always while supine)

0	No drift
1	Drift
2	Some effort vs gravity (leg drifts down to the bed)
3	No effort vs gravity
4	No movement
UN	Amputation or joint fusion

Test each leg in turn (nonparetic leg first). Drift is scored if a leg falls before 5 s. Score UN only for patients with amputations or joint fusions of the hip.

Fig. 3.2, cont'd

(Continued)

7. Limb ataxia **Ask patient (eyes open) to: "Touch your finger to your nose. Touch your heel to your shin"**	
0	Absent
1	Present in one limb
2	Present in two or more limbs
UN	Amputation or joint fusion
Perform finger-nose and heel-shin tests on both sides to determine unilateral cerebellar lesion. Score 0 for patients who are paralyzed or cannot understand. Score 1 or 2 only if ataxia is disproportionate to weakness. Score UN only for patients with amputations or joint fusions.	

8. Sensory **Test as many body parts as possible (arms [not hands], legs, trunk, face) for sensation using pinprick or noxious stimulus (in the obtunded or aphasic patient)**	
0	Normal
1	Mild-to-moderate sensory loss
2	Severe-to-total sensory loss
Score sensory loss due to stroke only. Stuporous and aphasic patients are scored 0 or 1. Patients with brain stem stroke and bilateral sensory loss, quadriplegic patients who do not respond, and comatose patients (item 1a = 3) are scored 2. A score of 2 is only given when a severe or total sensory loss is demonstrated.	

Fig. 3.2, cont'd

9. Best language
Using pictures and a sentence list (see reverse), ask the patient to: "Describe what you see in this picture. Name the items in this picture. Read these sentences"

0	No aphasia
1	Mild-to-moderate aphasia
2	Severe aphasia
3	Mute, global aphasia

Patients with visual loss can be asked to identify and describe objects placed in the hand. Intubated patients should be asked to write their answers. The examiner must choose a score for stuporous or uncooperative patients. Comatose patients (item 1a = 3) are scored 3. A score of 3 is only given if the patient is mute and unable to follow one-step commands.

10. Dysarthria
Using a simple word list (see reverse), ask the patient to: "Read these words" or "repeat these words"

0	Normal articulation
1	Mild-to-moderate dysarthria
2	Severe dysarthria
UN	Intubated or other physical barriers

Patients with severe aphasia can be scored based on the clarity of articulation of their spontaneous speech. Score UN only for patients who are intubated or have other physical barriers to speech. Do not tell patients why they are being tested.

Fig. 3.2, cont'd

(Continued)

11. Extinction and inattention Sufficient information to determine these scores may have been obtained during the prior testing	
0	No abnormality
1	Visual, tactile, auditory, spatial, or personal inattention
2	Profound hemi-inattention or extinction to more than one modality

Lack of patient response and inattention may already be evident from the previous items. Score 0 if the patient has a severe visual loss preventing visual double simultaneous stimulation, but the response to cutaneous stimuli is normal, or if the patient has aphasia but does not appear to attend to both sides. The presence of visual spatial attention or anosognosia may also be evidence of abnormality.

Fig. 3.2, cont'd

(Continued)

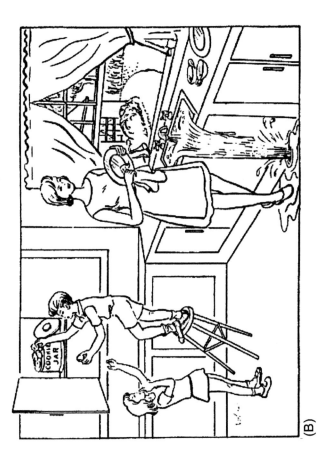

Fig. 3.2, cont'd   (B) cookie jar picture,

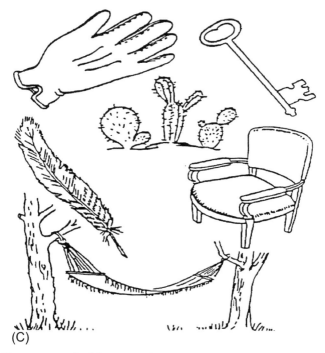

(C)

Fig. 3.2, cont'd   (C) NIHSS objects. (Reproduced from National Institute of Health, National Institute of Neurological Disorders and Stroke. Stroke Scale. https://www.coeuretavc.ca/-/media/pdf-files/canada/health-information-catalogue/hsf_strokeassessguide_v1_web_en.ashx, Copyright National Institute of Health.)

Ask the patient to repeat these words (assess for dysarthria):

MAMA

TIP-TOP

FIFTY-FIFTY

THANKS

HUCKLEBERRY

BASEBALL PLAYER

Ask the patient to read these sentences aloud:

You know how

Down to earth

I got home from work

Near the table in the dining room

They heard him speak on the radio last night

Aphasia and bedside language assessment

Aphasia is a disorder of language (spoken, written, or signed) that is acquired secondary to a brain injury. **Dysarthria** is a disorder of speech (articulation).

A patient with **Broca's aphasia** is nonfluent and omits small grammatical words. They have difficulty with naming, repetition, reading, writing, with intact comprehension (however detailed testing of comprehension can reveal some difficulty). It localizes to the inferior frontal gyrus in the dominant hemisphere.

A patient with **Wernicke's aphasia** is fluent, however, the content of speech is empty of meaning (paraphasias, neologisms, jargon). They have impaired naming, repetition, reading, and writing (which is very sensitive for Wernicke's). It localizes to the superior temporal gyrus in the dominant hemisphere.

We will briefly discuss the acute stroke bedside assessment for aphasia. There are six components to a language assessment: (1) **spontaneous speech** (fluency), (2) **comprehension**, (3) **naming**, (4) **repetition**, (5) **reading**, and (6) **writing**.

The fluency of speech, including paraphasic errors, word finding difficulties, and effort, can be assessed by open-ended questions and asking the patient to describe the cookie jar picture. Examples of paraphasic errors include phonemic (substitution of an incorrect sound; for example "shoon for spoon") or semantic (substitution of an incorrect word with related meaning; for example "knife for spoon").

Comprehension is assessed by the LOC commands part of the NIHSS (asking patient to "open and close your eyes, grip and release your hand"), and can be supplemented with additional questions to see if patients can consistently follow simple or complex instructions, e.g. try yes/no questions and pointing commands (touch your nose, point to the ceiling, touch your right ear with your left thumb, etc.). Naming and reading are assessed with the NIHSS naming cards and asking them to read the standard sentences. Repetition and writing are generally not assessed as part of the NIHSS but can be useful to evaluate. Ask patients to repeat sentences. Impairment in repetition is a sensitive indicator of aphasia.

We will now review pitfalls that may occur when scoring the NIHSS. Common ("tricky") scenarios often occur when scoring the NIHSS that are not explicit in the scoring system and often not taught when learning the NIHSS. Below we will illustrate the correct way to score these specific examples, along with practical tips.

1.1 How to score dysarthria in a patient that is aphasic?

<u>Answer</u>: If the patient is completely mute then they arbitrarily receive a score of 2 for dysarthria. However, if the patient is aphasic but able to verbalize, and there is no clear dysarthria, then they receive a score of 0.

1.2 How do I assess visual fields if the patient is not able to reliably communicate?

<u>Answer</u>: Firstly, our goal is to assess for gross visual field abnormalities. Try not to get bogged down by spending too much time on this bedside assessment in the code stroke setting. In a patient that is not able to communicate, use visual threat. Approach each visual field quadrant quickly with your hand and watch for the blink reflex (careful not to hit the eye). The absence of blink to threat on its own has a low specificity.

1.3 How do I score ataxia if the patient is weak?

<u>Answer</u>: The answer is the ataxia needs to be out of proportion to the degree of muscle weakness (easier said than done as this distinction comes with experience). Someone who is weak will be slow and may appear clumsy and mildly uncoordinated but should not be ataxic or have dysmetria on finger-to-nose or heel-to-shin examination. Ataxia is absent in the patient who cannot understand or is paralyzed.

Weakness and ataxia can coexist (e.g., ataxic–hemiparesis lacunar stroke syndrome). Make sure to have patient fully extend the arm to reach for the target; if the finger target is too close to the patient, you may miss the end-point dysmetria. The examiner can supplement finger-nose testing by asking the patient to perform the rapid hand tapping test (rhythmic tapping like a steady drum beat) and the rapid alternating hand movement test (alternating fist and palm), to assess for slowing (expected with limb paresis) or ataxia (irregular rhythm and force of the movements).

1.4 How do I assess the sensory examination if the patient cannot communicate?

<u>Answer</u>: The sensory examination should be done with a sharp object (i.e., a sterile safety pin or broken tongue depressor). You are looking for grimace/withdrawal in the patient that is obtunded or aphasic. A clinical pearl is to test the proximal area of the lower limb, as older people may have a length-dependent polyneuropathy (for many reasons, such as diabetes) at baseline affecting the distal limb.

1.5 How do I assess for neglect?

<u>Answer</u>: The parietal lobes are involved in spatial awareness. Lesions in the nondominant parietal lobe (i.e., right parietal lobe in the majority of patients) may lead to

inattention and extinction of the contralateral side. Other localizations include the right frontal lobe and thalamus.

Inattention (or neglect) occurs when patients ignore visual, somatosensory or auditory stimuli on the contralateral side, but may recognize it if their attention is strongly drawn there. This is not due to a primary sensory or motor abnormality. In severe cases, patients may fail to recognize their own limb. In extinction, when a stimulus is presented simultaneously with an identical stimulus on the unaffected side, the patient will neglect the contralateral stimulus. You cannot test extinction if the patient has a significant primary sensory modality loss. To test for tactile sensory extinction, ask the patient to close their eyes and tell you if you are touching the right hand, left hand, or both at the same time.

1.6 How do I distinguish visual extinction from a visual field deficit?

Answer: With a visual field deficit, any visual stimuli presented in that area will not be seen by the patient. With visual extinction, when a patient is presented with stimuli on both sides of the visual field they will neglect the contralateral stimulus, however, presenting stimuli *only* in the contralateral side will be appreciated. Turning the head in the direction of the deficit or cueing may ameliorate neglect but will not alter a homonymous visual field defect. You can also test for sensory extinction to other modalities (tactile and auditory).

Miscellaneous physical examination pearls

❑ Delirious patients will have fluctuations in attention or consciousness and should not make paraphasic errors, whereas stroke patients with isolated aphasia are usually attentive and trying to respond and often make paraphasic errors.

(Continued)

❏ Truncal and gait ataxia, a posterior circulation sign, is not assessed on the NIHSS, so a cerebellar stroke could potentially be missed if you do not check balance and gait. Therefore, do not forget to check to see if the patient can sit, stand, and walk normally if a cerebellar stroke is suspected. A clinical pearl is that if a patient can walk normally, and especially if tandem gait is intact, then it is unlikely that the patient has a midline acute cerebellar lesion.

❏ Blood pressure is usually elevated in acute stroke (both ischemic and hemorrhagic) because of auto-regulation of cerebral perfusion pressure.

What clues on physical examination suggest a functional (psychogenic) disorder?

Diagnosis of a psychogenic (nonorganic or functional) disorder can be difficult even for experienced clinicians. This is *always* a diagnosis of exclusion, particularly in the acute stroke setting. Some patients may have functional overlay or exaggerated illness behavior that is superimposed on genuine stroke deficits.

Give-way weakness, variable weakness, and non-anatomical patterns

❏ Initially, the patient displays full or reasonable power in the affected limb but it then gives-way or collapses when resistance is applied. False positives can occur when the patient has pain or does not understand the instructions.

❏ Also look for inconsistency in responses (variability in weakness upon repeated testing and in different positions, e.g. supine, seated, walking), weakness that does not fit a typical upper motor neuron pattern or anatomical distribution of muscle groups affected, and suggestibility.

Co-contraction

❏ The antagonist muscle contracts when testing the agonist muscle group. For example, you feel the triceps contracting when testing elbow flexion (biceps).

Hoover's sign

❏ The patient attempts to flex the "weak" leg at the hip, while the examiner feels for extension of the unaffected leg. If the patient has a functional weakness the unaffected leg will not push down onto the bed (effort is not being transmitted to the other leg). Again, beware of false positives from pain, neglect, or poor understanding of directions.

Splitting of the midline sensation loss

❏ Anatomically, the demarcation of sensory loss in the trunk is not perfectly midline as a result of overlapping innervation from the contralateral intercostal nerves.

Waxy flexibility

❏ A sign of catatonia
❏ When the patient's arm is held against gravity and released, it maintains position and does not dropdown.

Guarding of hand dropping over face

❏ Raise the hand above the face. It avoids the face when dropped when presumably there is flaccid weakness.

How to make sense of unusual signs on physical examination

Right-/wrong-way eyes:

Right-way eyes occur in lesions affecting the *frontal eye fields*. The frontal eye fields normally aid in contralateral eye movements, however when there is injury (from ischemia for example), then the eyes look toward the side of the lesion (i.e., away from the hemiparetic side).

(Continued)

Wrong-way eyes look toward the side of the weakness and away from the side of the lesion. Causes include:

❑ Seizure activity in the cortex, which causes activation (rather than damage) of the frontal eye fields.

❑ For unclear reasons, thalamic hemorrhage can disrupt the corticospinal pathways of the internal capsule leading to contralateral weakness and also cause wrong-way eyes (these thalamic lesions are typically large and usually accompanied by deep coma).

❑ Lesions in the pontine basis and tegmentum disrupt the corticospinal fibers leading to contralateral hemiplegia, with the involvement of the sixth nerve nucleus (or PPRF) causing ipsilateral horizontal gaze palsy.

Diaphoresis, confusion, pale skin

❑ Suggests hypoglycemia or other metabolic abnormality or presyncope.

Pupils

❑ Dilated pupils suggest a sympathomimetic toxidrome (amphetamines, cocaine, pseudoephedrine, cholinergic antagonist drugs, etc.).

❑ Constricted pupils suggest opioid or narcotic overdose. Pontine tegmental injury typically results in pinpoint pupils. The most common cause is pontine hemorrhage.

❑ Lesions in the lateral medullary tegmentum (Wallenberg's syndrome) may cause an ipsilateral Horner's syndrome.

Sensory level (without cranial nerve deficits)

❑ Localizes to the spinal cord.

Before we move on to stroke syndromes and code stroke imaging, here is a clinical code stroke algorithm that summarizes the first part of the code stroke—starting from when the ED/stroke team is alerted of a code stroke, to just prior to stroke imaging (Fig. 3.3). Later in the book, we will review an imaging code stroke algorithm.

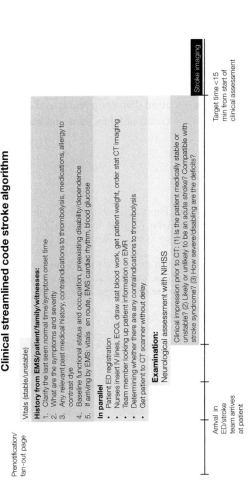

Clinical streamlined code stroke algorithm

Prenotification/fan-out page

Vitals (stable/unstable)

History from EMS/patient/family/witnesses:
1. Clarify the last seen normal time/symptom onset time
2. What are the symptoms and severity
3. Any relevant past medical history, contraindications to thrombolysis, medications, allergy to contrast dye
4. Baseline functional status and occupation, preexisting disability/dependence
5. If arriving by EMS: vitals en route, EMS cardiac rhythm, blood glucose

In parallel
- Patient ED registration
- Nurses insert IV lines, ECG, draw stat blood work, get patient weight, order stat CT imaging
- Team member looking up patient information on EMR
- Determining whether there are any contraindications to thrombolysis
- Get patient to CT scanner without delay

Examination:
Neurological assessment with NIHSS

Clinical impression prior to CT: (1) Is the patient medically stable or unstable? (2) Likely or unlikely to be an acute stroke? Compatible with stroke syndrome? (3) How severe/disabling are the deficits?

Stroke imaging

Arrival in ED/stroke team arrives at patient

Target time <15 min from start of clinical assessment

Fig. 3.3   Clinical streamlined code stroke algorithm. The code stroke starts with the EMS prenotification or fan-out page. There are many tasks that are completed in parallel and sequential that ends with the clinical impression prior to stroke imaging. The target time from when the clinical assessment starts to the first CT scan slice is less than 15 min.

Summary

In this chapter, we reviewed the NIHSS and the common "tricky" scoring and clinical scenarios with practical clinical tips. When you are under time pressure, look for cortical signs early in the examination (aphasia, neglect, gaze deviation)—this can be a tip-off to the presence of a large vessel occlusion, which has implications for activating the endovascular team. We also discussed different physical examination maneuvers that are associated with functional disorders and stroke mimics.

Further Reading

1. Abdelnour LH, El-Nagi F. Functional neurological disorder presenting as stroke: a narrative review. *J Psychol Abnorm*. 2017;6:1.

2. Blumenfeld H. *Neuroanatomy Through Clinical Cases*. 2nd ed. Oxford University Press; 2010.

3. Boulanger JM, et al. Canadian stroke best practice recommendations for acute stroke management: prehospital, emergency department, and acute inpatient stroke care, 6th edition, update 2018. *Int J Stroke*. 2018;13(9):949–984.

4. Caplan L. *Caplan's Stroke. A Clinical Approach*. 4th ed. Boston: Elsevier Canada; 2009.

5. Liberman A, Prabhakaran S. Stroke chameleons and stroke mimics in the emergency department. *Curr Neurol Neurosci Rep*. 2017;17(2):15.

6. National Institute of Health, National Institute of Neurological Disorders and Stroke. *Stroke Scale*. https://www.coeuretavc.ca/-/media/pdf-files/canada/health-information-catalogue/hsf_strokeassessguide_v1_web_en.ashx.

7. Stone J, Sharpe M. Hoover's sign. *Pract Neurol*. 2001;1:50–53.

CHAPTER 4

Stroke syndromes

This chapter is the cornerstone of acute stroke. In contrast to general neurology where neurologists ask, "where is the lesion and what is the lesion?" the correlate question of stroke neurology becomes, "what is the vascular territory involved and what is the vascular lesion?"

The famous quote by C. Miller Fisher is that "*neurology is learned stroke by stroke.*"

This chapter provides an approach to the common (and uncommon) clinical stroke syndromes with associated neuroanatomical figures. The most common stroke syndromes are highlighted in these pink colored boxes. Readers interested in these more common presentations, or those who are just starting out on a stroke rotation or neurology residency, may focus their reading on the neuroanatomical figures and the pink colored boxes. Experienced readers interested in a review of common and uncommon stroke syndromes would benefit from reading the entire chapter.

This chapter is not meant to be a comprehensive review of cerebral and vascular anatomy. However, here are some high-yield diagrams (Figs. 4.1–4.3) that may be helpful to review before reading through the different clinical stroke syndromes.

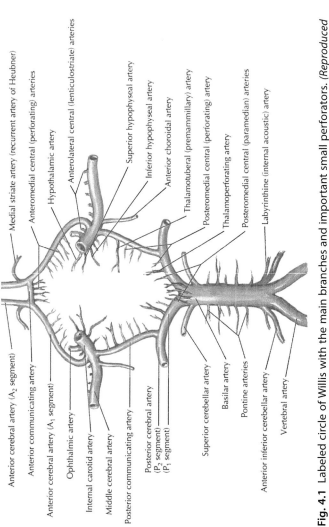

Anterior cerebral artery (A₂ segment)

Anterior communicating artery

Anterior cerebral artery (A₁ segment)

Ophthalmic artery

Internal carotid artery

Middle cerebral artery

Posterior communicating artery

Posterior cerebral artery
(P₂ segment)
(P₁ segment)

Superior cerebellar artery

Basilar artery

Pontine arteries

Anterior inferior cerebellar artery

Vertebral artery

Medial striate artery (recurrent artery of Heubner)

Anteromedial central (perforating) arteries

Hypothalamic artery

Anterolateral central (lenticulostriate) arteries

Superior hypophyseal artery

Inferior hypophyseal artery

Anterior choroidal artery

Thalamotuberal (premammillary) artery

Posteromedial central (perforating) artery

Thalamoperforating artery

Posteromedial central (paramedian) arteries

Labyrinthine (internal acoustic) artery

Fig. 4.1 Labeled circle of Willis with the main branches and important small perforators. *(Reproduced with permission from Felten D, Maida M, Netter F, O'Banion M. Netter's Atlas of Neuroscience. 3rd ed. Canada: Elsevier; 2015, Copyright (2015) Elsevier Canada.)*

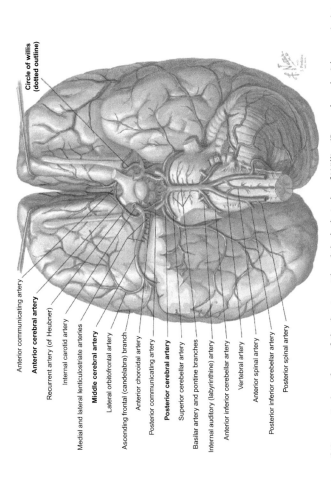

Anterior communicating artery

Anterior cerebral artery

Recurrent artery (of Heubner)

Internal carotid artery

Medial and lateral lenticulostriate arteries

Middle cerebral artery

Lateral orbitofrontal artery

Ascending frontal (candelabra) branch

Anterior choroidal artery

Posterior communicating artery

Posterior cerebral artery

Superior cerebellar artery

Basilar artery and pontine branches

Internal auditory (labyrinthine) artery

Anterior inferior cerebellar artery

Vertebral artery

Anterior spinal artery

Posterior inferior cerebellar artery

Posterior spinal artery

Circle of willis (dotted outline)

Fig. 4.2 A view of the ventral surface of the brain with a labeled circle of Willis. *(Reproduced with permission from Felten D, Maida M, Netter F, O'Banion M. Netter's Atlas of Neuroscience. 3rd ed. Canada: Elsevier; 2015, Copyright (2015) Elsevier Canada.)*

Clinical pearl: Textbook circle of Willis anatomy is only seen approximately 25% of the time.

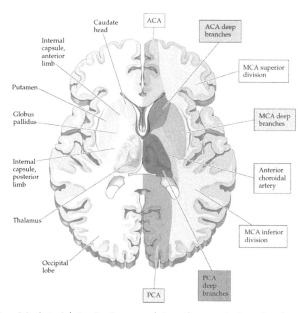

Fig. 4.3 Arterial territories supplying the cortical and subcortical brain regions. *(Reproduced with permission from Blumenfeld H. Neuroanatomy Through Clinical Cases. 2nd ed. Oxford University Press; 2010, Copyright (2010) Oxford University Press.)*

Below is an outline and approach to the different stroke syndromes. A clinical pearl is to remember to ask handedness as it is important in determining hemispheric dominance.

Approach to Stroke Syndromes

Large vessel disease

<u>Anterior circulation</u>
Middle cerebral artery
- Complete left and right MCA syndromes, partial syndromes, and Gerstmann syndrome

Anterior cerebral artery
- Complete left and right ACA syndromes, partial syndromes, and Recurrent Artery of Heubner

Anterior choroidal artery

<u>Posterior circulation</u>
Basilar artery
- Proximal and top of the basilar syndromes

Posterior cerebral artery
- Complete left and right PCA syndromes and Balint syndrome

Small vessel disease (Lacunar syndromes)
Pure motor
Pure sensory
Mixed sensorimotor
Ataxic hemiparesis
Dysarthria-clumsy hand

Brainstem
Lateral and medial medullary syndrome
Pontine syndromes (four)
Midbrain syndromes (three)

Spinal cord
Anterior and posterior spinal artery syndrome

Thalamic syndromes

1 ANTERIOR CIRCULATION

The anterior circulation originates (as seen in Fig. 4.4) from the common carotid artery (CCA). In typical anatomy, the right CCA originates from the brachiocephalic

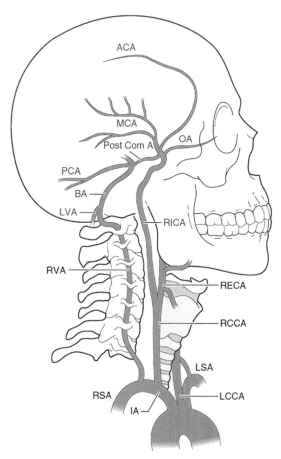

Fig. 4.4 A view from the right extracranial cerebral-bound arteries. *ACA*, anterior cerebral artery; *BA*, basilar artery; *IA*, innominate artery; *LCCA/RCCA*, left/right common carotid artery; *LSA/RSA*, left/right subclavian artery; *LVA/RVA*, left/right vertebral artery; *MCA*, middle cerebral artery; *OA*, ophthalmic artery; *PCA*, posterior cerebral artery; *Post Com A*, posterior communicating artery; *RECA*, right external carotid artery; *RICA*, right internal carotid artery. *(Reproduced with permission from Grotta J, et al. Stroke: Pathophysiology, Diagnosis, and Management. 6th ed. Canada: Elsevier; 2015, Copyright (2015) Elsevier Canada.)*

trunk and the left CCA originates from the aortic arch. The CCA bifurcates approximately at the level of C6 into the internal carotid artery (ICA) and the external carotid artery (ECA). We will focus on the ICA as it is responsible for the cerebral anterior circulation.

There are seven segments of the ICA:

(1) Cervical
(2) Petrous
(3) Lacerum
(4) Cavernous
(5) Clinoid
(6) Ophthalmic (supraclinoid)
(7) Communicating (terminal)

The ophthalmic artery is the first major branch of the ICA, as it pierces the dura. Another clinically relevant branch off the ICA is the anterior choroidal artery.

The ICA then bifurcates into the anterior cerebral artery and the middle cerebral artery. See Figs. 4.5 and 4.6.

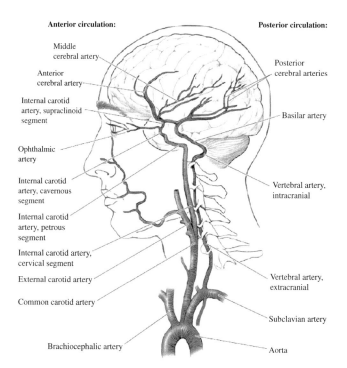

Fig. 4.5 Important branches/segments of the internal carotid artery. *(Reproduced with permission from Blumenfeld H. Neuroanatomy Through Clinical Cases. 2nd ed. Oxford University Press; 2010, Copyright (2010) Oxford University Press.)*

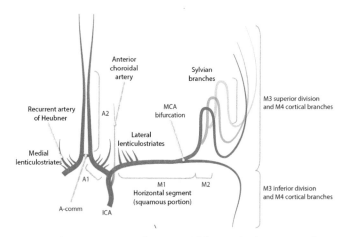

Fig. 4.6 The anterior circulation—middle cerebral artery and anterior cerebral artery; both branches of the internal carotid artery. *(Reproduced with permission from Mandell J. Core Radiology. Cambridge University Press; 2013, Copyright (2013) Cambridge University Press.)*

1.1 Middle cerebral artery

The most common artery affected in ischemic stroke is the middle cerebral artery (MCA). The different segments, branches, and patterns of infarction can be seen in Fig. 4.7. We will review each pattern.

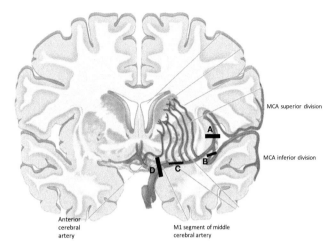

MCA superior division

MCA inferior division

Anterior
cerebral
artery

M1 segment of middle
cerebral artery

Fig. 4.7 Coronal view of the branches of the middle cerebral artery with different patterns of infarction. The *black* lines depict arterial occlusions at different locations. (A) Occlusion of the upper (superior) trunk of the MCA, (B) occlusion of the lower (inferior) trunk of the MCA, (C) infarct of the deep basal ganglia (i.e., junctional plaque), and (D) occlusion of the proximal MCA (M1 segment). *(Reproduced and edited with permission from Blumenfeld H. Neuroanatomy Through Clinical Cases. 2nd ed. Oxford University Press; 2010, Copyright (2010) Oxford University Press.)*

Below we will describe the stroke syndromes associated with occlusion of the above divisions of the MCA.

1.1.1 Occlusion of the upper trunk of the MCA

The upper trunk supplies the frontal and superior parietal lobes. The neurological symptoms associated with this syndrome include:

❏ Contralateral hemiparesis face and upper extremity with relative sparing of the lower extremity

- This is a result of the lateral aspect of the motor homunculus being affected where the face and arm are represented
❏ Contralateral hemisensory loss, sometimes sparing the leg
❏ Contralateral inferior quadrantanopia
❏ Conjugate ipsilateral eye deviation
  - The frontal eye fields are located in the frontal cortex and are responsible for voluntary eye movements toward the contralateral direction. Infarction affecting the frontal eye fields results in the eyes "falling" toward the side of the lesion (the eyes look away from the hemiplegic side). That is, there is either a partial or a complete gaze paresis on attempting to look toward the lesion (or away from the hemiplegia).

<u>Nondominant hemisphere</u>:
❏ Inattention/neglect of the contralateral side of space. Visual, somatosensory, and auditory modalities can be affected
  - The right hemisphere is thought to be more important in attentional mechanisms (lesions in left hemisphere cause mild or undetectable attentional deficits). This is because the right hemisphere attends to both left and right-sided stimuli, but more strongly to stimuli on the left, whereas the left hemisphere only attends to stimuli on the right side
  - Hemispatial neglect, defined as a deficit in attention to and awareness of one side of the field of vision can be observed. The neglect of input, or "inattention," includes ignoring contralesional sights, sounds, or tactile stimuli

❏ Anosognosia, which is a lack of insight into the neurological deficits

❏ Asomatognosia, which is a loss of recognition or awareness of a part of the body on the left side

<u>Dominant hemisphere</u>:

❏ Aphasia (Broca's)

- Broca's area is located in the inferior frontal gyrus

❏ Apraxia—such as ideomotor apraxia, which is an inability to perform purposeful motor movements that cannot be attributed to a primary sensorimotor deficit. There are many forms of apraxia that are beyond the scope of this book. Ask the patient to pantomime brushing their teeth or combing their hair

1.1.2   Occlusion of the inferior trunk of the MCA

The inferior trunk supplies the lateral surface of the temporal lobe and inferior parietal lobe. This can be a difficult clinical localization to identify at the bedside. The neurological symptoms associated with this syndrome include:

❏ No motor or sensory abnormalities

- The primary motor and sensory cortex are not affected

❏ Contralateral superior quadrantanopia

- Visual pathway (Meyer's loop) runs through the lower aspect of the temporal lobe

❏ May be irascible, paranoid or violent, and mistaken for delirium

<u>Nondominant hemisphere</u>:

❏ Often agitated, hyperactive state resembling delirium

<u>Dominant hemisphere</u>:

❑ Aphasia (Wernicke's)
- Wernicke's area is located in the inferior parietal/superior temporal lobe

1.1.3 Infarct of the deep basal ganglia (junctional plaque)

This results from stenosis or occlusion of the main stem MCA before or across its lenticulostriate branches. This should not be confused with infarcts from small vessel disease (i.e., lacunes, which we will discuss later in the chapter). These may be seen in isolation as collateral circulation may be adequate to prevent extensive cortical infarction. These lesions are larger than lacunes and often extend to the inferior brain surface. These are often termed <u>junctional plaque</u> or <u>branch artery occlusion</u>. The neurological symptoms associated with this syndrome include:

❑ Contralateral hemiparesis
❑ Sensory loss is usually minor
- This is a result of sparing of the thalamus/posterior limb the internal capsule

<u>Nondominant hemisphere</u>:
❑ Inattention/neglect of contralateral side of space (more transient than with parietal cortical infarction)

<u>Dominant hemisphere</u>:
❑ After a short period of temporary mutism, speech is sparse and dysarthric, with sparing of repetition (similar to transcortical aphasia)

1.1.4 Occlusion of distal MCA branch

The etiology is almost always embolic and the syndrome will depend on the distal branch affected.

1.1.5 Occlusion of the proximal MCA segment (M1 segment)

Proximal middle cerebral artery syndrome (i.e., occlusion of M1)

This results from occlusion of the proximal, or M1 segment of the MCA: *an ideal target for endovascular treatment.* The neurological symptoms associated with this syndrome include:

❏ Contralateral hemiplegia (upper extremity > lower extremity)
❏ Hemisensory loss
❏ Conjugate eye deviation (looking toward the side of the lesion)
❏ Contralateral hemianopia

<u>Nondominant hemisphere</u>:

❏ Hemispatial neglect
❏ Anosognosia
❏ Drowsiness and eyelid opening apraxia (less commonly seen)

<u>Dominant hemisphere</u>:

❏ Global aphasia
❏ Apraxia (ideomotor apraxia for example)

1.1.6 Other MCA syndromes
Gerstmann syndrome

This uncommon stroke syndrome results from ischemia/infarction to the dominant inferior parietal lobe, in the region of the angular gyrus. There is a tetrad of neurological symptoms associated with this syndrome, which include:

 (i) Agraphia (impairment in writing)
 (ii) Acalculia (impairment in arithmetic)
(iii) Left–right disorientation
(iv) Finger agnosia (difficulty naming or identifying individual fingers)

This syndrome usually is accompanied by other deficits resulting from a larger lesion involving the dominant parietal lobe. Accompanying symptoms include a contralateral visual field deficit, alexia, anomia, or more significant aphasia.

1.2 Anterior cerebral artery

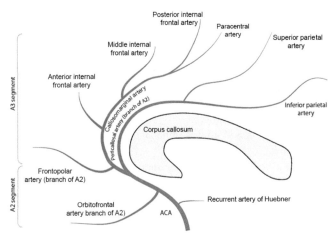

Fig. 4.8 Anterior cerebral artery and its distal branches. *(Reproduced with permission from Mandell J. Core Radiology. Cambridge University Press; 2013, Copyright (2013) Cambridge University Press.)*

The anterior cerebral artery (ACA) and its distal branches are illustrated in Fig. 4.8. ACA strokes are much less common than MCA infarcts. They often occur in conjunction with MCA infarction in the setting of a proximal occlusion (i.e., carotid "T" occlusion). As well, the pattern of infarction is simpler than the MCA. The single most important clinical cue of an ACA-territory infarction is the distribution of weakness. Typically, there is leg > arm weakness.

Anterior cerebral artery syndrome

The neurological symptoms associated with this syndrome include:

❏ Contralateral leg weakness and/or sensory loss (may be present and mild in the contralateral leg)
❏ Contralateral motor neglect
❏ Incontinence (especially in bilateral lesions)
❏ "Alien hand sign" (frontal variant)—involuntary movement of the hand (one hand acts against the other or acts involuntarily). This is from the involvement of the mesial frontal lobe and genu as well as the rostral body of the corpus callosum

<u>Nondominant hemisphere</u>:

❏ Acute confusional state

<u>Dominant hemisphere</u>:

❏ Transcortical motor aphasia (supplementary motor area)
❏ Contralateral ideomotor apraxia
   - involvement of the anterior corpus callosum, causing disconnection of the right sensorimotor cortex from language region in the left hemisphere and manifesting in impairment in the use of the left hand for writing
❏ Abulia (most often in bilateral infarction), which is a state of apathy, reduced spontaneous and limited quantity of speech and in its most severe form, mutism.

An anatomic variant in which the right and left ACAs stem from a common A1 trunk can result in bilateral ACA territory infarction. This clinically presents as sudden onset bilateral leg weakness (which can mimic a spinal cord lesion).

1.2.1 Occlusion of the recurrent artery of Heubner

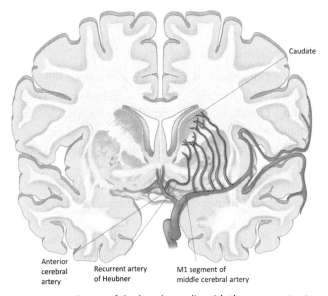

Fig. 4.9 Coronal view of the basal ganglia with the recurrent artery of Heubner, a branch off the ACA. *(Reproduced with permission from Blumenfeld H. Neuroanatomy Through Clinical Cases. 2nd ed. Oxford University Press; 2010, Copyright (2010) Oxford University Press.)*

The recurrent artery of Heubner is a branch of the ACA that supplies the caudate head and anterior limb of the internal capsule, seen in Fig. 4.9 (interesting fact: only 25% of individuals have a single artery of Heubner, the remainder have either two, three, or four recurrent arteries). The neurological symptoms associated with this syndrome include:

❏ Behavior changes (abulia, agitated, slowness of thought). Cognitive changes resemble lesions in the medial thalamus and frontal and temporal lobes.

❏ Contralateral hemiparesis (face, arm, and leg)

❏ Dysarthria
❏ Right caudate—restlessness and hyperactivity, and left visual neglect

1.3 Anterior choroidal artery

The anterior choroidal artery originates from the internal carotid artery (after the ophthalmic and posterior communicating branches). It supplies the globus pallidus, lateral geniculate body, posterior limb of the internal capsule, and medial temporal lobe. The neurological symptoms associated with this syndrome include:

❏ Contralateral hemiparesis (face, arm, and leg)
❏ Significant hemisensory loss (often temporary)
❏ Hemianopia
  - If the lateral geniculate nucleus (in the thalamus) is affected, can result in a homonymous hemianopia, quadrantanopsia, or sectoranopia (wedge-shaped visual defect)
❏ *Absence of persistent neglect, aphasia, or other cortical signs.

2 POSTERIOR CIRCULATION

Before we discuss posterior circulation syndromes, let us review the posterior circulation vascular supply (Figs. 4.10 and 4.11).

The vertebral arteries originate from the subclavian arteries on either side. The vertebral arteries travel through the transverse foramen of the cervical vertebral bodies and then pierce the dura to enter the intracranial cavity through the foramen magnum. They join together to form the basilar artery which travels along the anterior surface of the pons. The posterior inferior cerebral arteries (PICA) branch off the distal vertebral arteries prior to the basilar

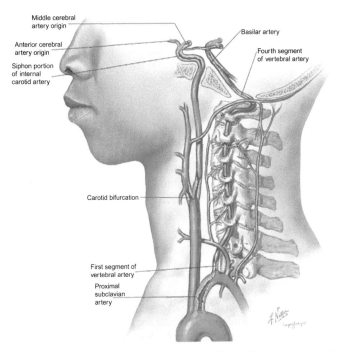

Fig. 4.10 Posterior circulation and sites with higher prevalence of atherosclerosis. *(Reproduced with permission from Felten D, Maida M, Netter F, O'Banion M. Netter's Atlas of Neuroscience. 3rd ed. Canada: Elsevier; 2015, Copyright (2015) Elsevier Canada.)*

artery and supply the posterior and inferior regions of the cerebellum and the dorsolateral aspect of the medulla. The anterior inferior cerebral arteries (AICA) arise from the proximal portion of the basilar artery and supply the basis pontis, lateral pontine tegmentum, flocculus, and anteroinferior portions of the cerebellum. The superior cerebellar arteries (SCA) branch from the distal basilar artery and supply the lateral pontine tegmentum and tectum of the mesencephalon and the superior vermis, lateral portion of the cerebellar hemispheres, and most of the cerebellar nuclei.

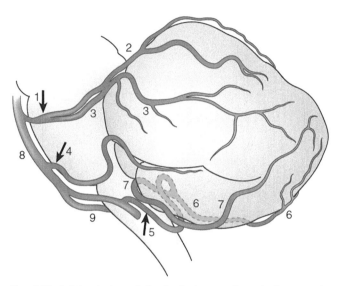

Fig. 4.11 A lateral view of the brainstem and cerebellar vascular supply. 1, Superior cerebellar artery (2, medial branch; 3, lateral branch); 4, anterior inferior cerebellar artery; 5, posterior inferior cerebellar artery (6, medial branch; 7, lateral branch); 8, basilar artery; 9, vertebral artery. *(Reproduced with permission from Grotta J, et al. Stroke: Pathophysiology, Diagnosis, and Management. 6th ed. Canada: Elsevier, 2015, Copyright (2015) Elsevier Canada.)*

The basilar artery branches into the posterior cerebral arteries (PCA) at the level of the cerebral peduncle. The PCAs then loop laterally and posteriorly around the midbrain supplying the medial temporal lobe, portions of the parietal lobe, and the occipital lobes. Perforators of the PCA supply the midbrain and thalamus (Fig. 4.2).

2.1 Occlusion of the basilar artery

Basilar artery occlusion (BAO) accounts for about 1% of all ischemic strokes and is a devastating stroke syndrome. Untreated, acute BAO has a very high case fatality and most survivors are left with severe disability, with some surviving in a tragic "locked-in" state (awake but quadriplegic, unable to speak, and ventilator-dependent). This is a syndrome that you do not want to miss, especially because the time window for potential treatment with tPA or endovascular therapy can be longer than it is for anterior circulation strokes. See Chapter 10 for further discussion of BAO and its treatment.

We will divide the syndrome into (i) proximal occlusion (Fig. 4.12) and (ii) top of the basilar syndrome (Fig. 4.13).

2.1.1 Proximal basilar artery occlusion

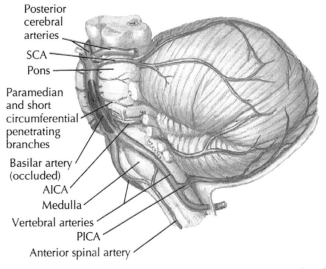

Fig. 4.12 Occlusion of the proximal basilar artery. *(Reproduced with permission from Felten D, Maida M, Netter F, O'Banion M. Netter's Atlas of Neuroscience. 3rd ed. Canada: Elsevier; 2015, Copyright (2015) Elsevier Canada.)*

This results in loss of perfusion to all upstream arteries including the paramedian basilar perforators supplying the pons, SCA, and PCA (although in some instances, the top of the basilar artery and PCAs can receive retrograde collateral flow from the anterior circulation via the posterior communicating arteries).

Proximal basilar artery syndrome

The neurological symptoms associated with this syndrome include:

❑ Altered LOC (hypersomnolent or coma)
❑ Quadriparesis or quadreplegia (may have asymmetry)
❑ May have a "crossed paralysis," i.e., right face and left limbs or vice versa
❑ May have abnormal movements such as jerking, tremor, twitching, and shivering. These movements may be misdiagnosed as seizure activity
❑ Oculomotor abnormalities; diplopia
  - These may include: <u>horizontal gaze palsy</u>, (complete or unilateral), unilateral or bilateral internuclear ophthalmoplegia (INO), one and a half syndrome, skew deviation, gaze paretic nystagmus, bilateral ptosis, among others
❑ Pupillary abnormalities
  - May have pinpoint pupils
❑ ataxia
❑ Bulbar symptoms (often bilateral)
  - These may include facial weakness, dysphagia, dysarthria, or dysphonia. Palatal myoclonus may be present
❑ Pseudobulbar affect

2.1.2 Top of the basilar syndrome

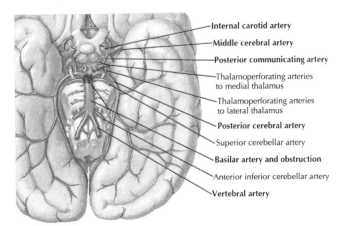

Fig. 4.13 Top of the basilar occlusion. *(Reproduced with permission from Felten D, Maida M, Netter F, O'Banion M. Netter's Atlas of Neuroscience. 3rd ed. Canada: Elsevier; 2015, Copyright (2015) Elsevier Canada.)*

This can result in ischemia/infarction of the midbrain, thalamus, and occipital lobes (sparing the pons).

The neurological symptoms associated with this syndrome include:

❏ Pupillary abnormalities (involvement of afferents to Edinger-Westphal nucleus, third nerve nucleus or descending sympathetic system)
– Pupils may be small, mid-position or dilated depending on the level and extent of the lesion
❏ Eye movement abnormalities
– <u>Vertical gaze impairment</u>
– Convergence-retraction nystagmus
❏ Altered LOC (hypersomnolent or coma)
❏ Amnesia
❏ Agitation, hallucinations (peduncular hallucinosis—vivid, visual, multiple colors, and objects)
❏ Homonymous hemianopia

2.2 Posterior cerebral artery

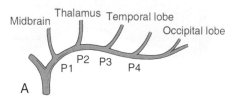

Fig. 4.14 Segments of the posterior cerebral artery and their parenchymal supply. *(Reproduced with permission from Grotta J, et al. Stroke: Pathophysiology, Diagnosis, and Management. 6th ed. Canada: Elsevier, 2015, Copyright (2015) Elsevier Canada.)*

The posterior cerebral artery has penetrating branches supplying the midbrain and thalamus (Fig. 4.14). It then branches to the occipital lobes and supplies the medial and inferior portions of the temporal lobes.

Posterior cerebral artery syndrome

The neurological symptoms associated with this syndrome include:

❏ Hemianopia
  - If the lower bank of the calcarine fissure is affected it results in a contralateral <u>superior</u> quadrantanopia. If the superior bank of the calcarine fissure is affected it results in a contralateral <u>inferior</u> quadrantanopia. If both are affected it results in complete homonymous hemianopia
❏ Concomitant visual inattention/neglect. This occurs when the parietal-occipital lobe is involved, predominantly on the right
❏ Contralateral hemisensory loss. If the thalamus is involved, specifically the ventroposterolateral nuclei (VPL)

❑ Contralateral hemiplegia (uncommon). If the mid-brain cerebral peduncle is affected

Dominant hemisphere:

❑ Alexia without agraphia. Infarction of the occipital lobe and the splenium of the corpus callosum (interrupts communication between the hemispheres). In this syndrome, patients can write but they cannot read. There may be an accompanying defect in color naming

❑ Difficulty in naming objects (transcortical sensory aphasia)

❑ Altered memory (anterograde amnesia). Occurs when the medial temporal lobes are involved

❑ Visual agnosia. When presented with an object, they have difficulty verbally describing what an object is used for. If they have sensory cues by placing the object in the hand, they can often correctly identify it

Nondominant hemisphere:

❑ Prosopagnosia (difficulty recognizing familiar faces; even their own face in a mirror)

Bilateral hemisphere:

❑ Cortical blindness (termed Anton syndrome). Often patients will confabulate what they see

Balint syndrome

This syndrome results from bilateral infarction of the parietal-occipital lobes (watershed area between MCA and PCA territory), often from hypoperfusion seen with significant hypotension or blood loss perioperatively. The neurological symptoms associated with this syndrome include:

❏ Simultanagnosia: the inability to see all the objects in the visual field (i.e., integrate an entire visual scene) at one time and may notice only parts of the objects, despite normal visual acuity

❏ Optic ataxia: the inability to accurately coordinate eye and hand movements

❏ Ocular apraxia: inability to voluntarily direct gaze accurately toward a target

3 LACUNAR SYNDROMES

A lacune is a small infarct, typically defined as less than 1.5 cm. There are many different clinical lacunar syndromes, five of which are clinically relevant and usually associated with small vessel cerebrovascular disease. Lacunar infarcts typically result from occlusion of a small penetrating branch artery (Fig. 4.15) most often related to chronic hypertensive lipohyalinosis but some may be embolic. From a general anatomic perspective, these syndromes can result from ischemia/infarction anywhere from the basis pontis up to the centrum semiovale. The most common locations include lentiform nucleus (putamen and globus pallidus), pons, thalamus, caudate, posterior limb of the internal capsule, and corona radiata. These syndromes lack cortical signs such as aphasia, agnosia, neglect, apraxia, visual field defects, as well as loss of consciousness and seizures.

Below we will describe the most common lacunar syndromes, their localization, and vascular supply. Lacunar stroke may present acutely or may have a gradually progressive or fluctuating onset over many hours.

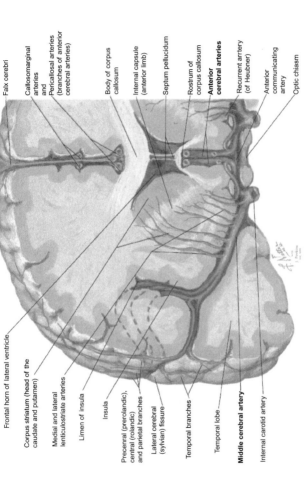

Falx cerebri

Callosomarginal arteries and

Pericallosal arteries (branches of anterior cerebral arteries)

Body of corpus callosum

Internal capsule (anterior limb)

Septum pellucidum

Rostrum of corpus callosum

Anterior cerebral arteries

Recurrent artery (of Heubner)

Anterior communicating artery

Optic chiasm

Frontal horn of lateral ventricle

Corpus striatum (head of the caudate and putamen)

Medial and lateral lenticulostriate arteries

Limen of insula

Insula

Precentral (prerolandic), central (rolandic) and parietal branches

Lateral cerebral (sylvian) fissure

Temporal branches

Temporal lobe

Middle cerebral artery

Internal carotid artery

Fig. 4.15 A coronal view of the lenticulostriate penetrating arteries of the proximal middle cerebral artery. (Reproduced with permission from Felten D, Maida M, Netter F, O'Banion M. Netter's Atlas of Neuroscience. 3rd ed. Canada: Elsevier; 2015, Copyright (2015) Elsevier Canada.)

Common lacunar syndromes

Pure motor

This is the most common lacunar syndrome, accounting for approximately 50% of all lacunar syndromes. It results in contralateral face/arm/leg weakness, in the absence of sensory or cortical signs. The homunculus is preserved in a compact somatotopic arrangement in the posterior limb of the internal capsule, therefore lesions in this location often produce weakness of the <u>entire</u> contralateral body (face, arm, and leg are typically affected equally), compared to a lesion affecting the MCA which typically involves face and arm ≫ leg.

Localization:

❏ Posterior limb of the internal capsule, corona radiata, and basis pontis

Vascular supply:

❏ Lenticulostriate branches from the MCA or basilar perforators

Pure sensory

This syndrome results in face/arm/leg sensory signs in the contralateral side of the body, in the absence of motor, or cortical signs.

Localization:

❏ Thalamus (VPM/VPL), corona radiata

Vascular supply:

❏ Lenticulostriate branches from the MCA or thalamoperforators from the PCA

Mixed sensorimotor

This localization results in contralateral face, arm, and leg weakness and sensory signs, with the absence of cortical signs.

Localization:
❑ Thalamocapsular, lateral pons

Vascular supply:
❑ Lenticulostriate branches from the MCA or PCA, or basilar perforators

Dysarthria–clumsy hand

This is the least common lacunar syndrome and results in facial weakness, dysarthria and slight weakness/clumsiness of the contralateral hand. There are no associated sensory or cortical signs.

Localization:
❑ Corona radiata, anterior limb or genu of the internal capsule, basis pontis

Vascular supply:
❑ Lenticulostriate branches from the MCA or basilar perforators

Ataxic hemiparesis

This syndrome results in ipsilateral weakness (face, arm, and leg) and limb ataxia. The ataxia is out of proportion to the motor deficit. There are no associated sensory or cortical signs.

Localization:
❑ Posterior limb of the internal capsule, basis pontis, and corona radiata

Vascular supply:
❑ Lenticulostriate branches from the MCA or basilar perforators

4 BRAINSTEM SYNDROMES

The brainstem is supplied by the paramedian basilar branches and long circumferential branches, which are the AICA (anterior inferior cerebellar artery), PICA (posterior inferior cerebellar artery), and SCA (superior cerebellar artery). The motor (corticospinal) tract is paramedian and decussates at the level of the pyramids. A clinical pearl is that if the face has an upper motor neuron pattern weakness, the lesion has to be above the level of the mid pons where the seventh cranial nerve travels.

Below we will discuss the two main stroke syndromes of the medulla, four main syndromes of the pons, and three main syndromes of the midbrain. Depending on the size of the lesion, you may get all or a combination of the below symptoms.

Medullary stroke syndromes
  (i) Lateral medullary syndrome (Wallenberg syndrome)
 (ii) Medial medullary syndrome (Dejerine syndrome)

Pontine stroke syndromes
  (i) Inferior medial pontine syndrome (Foville syndrome)
 (ii) Inferior lateral pontine syndrome (Marie–Foix syndrome)
(iii) Medial mid-pontine syndrome
(iv) Lateral mid-pontine syndrome

Midbrain stroke syndromes

  (i) Midbrain peduncle (Weber syndrome)

 (ii) Dorsomedial midbrain (Claude syndrome)

(iii) Paramedian midbrain (Benedikt Syndrome)

    Rather than memorizing the symptoms associated with a particular syndrome, the rule of 4 in the brainstem is a helpful method to understand the anatomy of the brainstem and the associated vascular syndrome.

Rule of 4 in the brainstem

1. There are four cranial nerves in the **medulla** (9–12), four cranial nerves in the **pons** (5–8), and four cranial nerves **above the pons** (1–4).
2. There are four motor nuclei in midline and are divisible by 12 (3, 4, 6, 12).
3. There are four structures in the **MIDLINE** beginning with **M**:
   a. **M**otor pathway (contralateral corticospinal tract)
   b. **M**edial lemniscus (contralateral vibration and proprioception)
   c. **M**edial longitudinal fasciculus (ipsilateral internuclear ophthalmoplegia)
   d. **M**otor nuclei (ipsilateral loss of cranial nerve affected)
4. There are four structures to the side beginning with **S**:
   a. **S**pinocerebellar pathways (ipsilateral ataxia of arm and leg)
   b. **S**pinothalamic pathway (contralateral pain and temperature)
   c. **S**ensory nucleus of CN 5 (ipsilateral pain and temperature on the face)
   d. **S**ympathetic pathway (ipsilateral Horner's syndrome)

Try to apply this rule to the brainstem syndromes discussed below.

Gates P. The rule of 4 of the brainstem: a simplified method for understanding brainstem anatomy and brainstem vascular syndromes for the non-neurologist. Int Med J. 2005;35:263–266.

Lateral medullary syndrome

The vascular supply interrupted in a lateral medullary syndrome is the vertebral artery, and less likely the PICA. The neurological symptoms associated with this syndrome include (Fig 4.16):

❑ Ipsilateral ataxia, vertigo, nystagmus, and nausea. This results from the involvement of the inferior cerebellar peduncle and vestibular nuclei. This is often the most disabling clinical feature of this condition.

❑ Ipsilateral facial decreased pain and temperature sense. This is from the involvement of the trigeminal nucleus and tract.

❑ Contralateral arm/leg decreased pain and temperature sense. This is from spinothalamic tract involvement.

❑ Ipsilateral Horner's syndrome. The descending sympathetic fibers run in the lateral medulla.

❑ Hoarseness, dysphagia. This is from the involvement of the nucleus ambiguus. There is often a decreased gag reflex on the side of the lesion.

❑ Ipsilateral decreased taste. This is a result of nucleus solitarius involvement.

Importantly, there is no weakness associated with this syndrome. There is associated weakness only if the infarct extends more medially with the involvement of the pyramidal tract resulting in contralateral weakness.

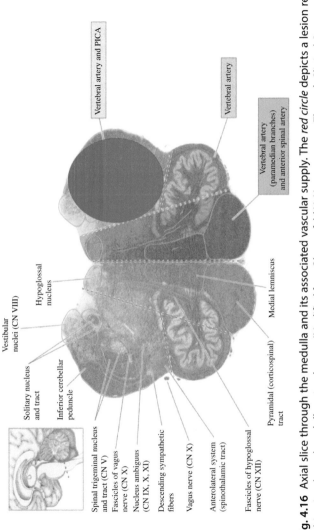

Fig. 4.16 Axial slice through the medulla and its associated vascular supply. The *red circle* depicts a lesion resulting in a lateral medullary syndrome. (Modified from Blumenfeld H. *Neuroanatomy Through Clinical Cases. 2nd ed.* Oxford University Press; 2010, Copyright (2010) Oxford University Press.)

Labels (clockwise):
- Vertebral artery and PICA
- Vertebral artery
- Vertebral artery (paramedian branches) and anterior spinal artery
- Medial lemniscus
- Pyramidal (corticospinal) tract
- Fascicles of hypoglossal nerve (CN XII)
- Anterolateral system (spinothalamic tract)
- Vagus nerve (CN X)
- Descending sympathetic fibers
- Nucleus ambiguus (CN IX, X, XI)
- Fascicles of vagus nerve (CN X)
- Spinal trigeminal nucleus and tract (CN V)
- Inferior cerebellar peduncle
- Solitary nucleus and tract
- Vestibular nuclei (CN VIII)
- Hypoglossal nucleus

4.1 Medial medullary syndrome

This syndrome (Fig. 4.17) results from occlusion of the paramedian branches of the anterior spinal artery or the vertebral artery. The neurological symptoms associated with this syndrome include:

❏ Contralateral arm/leg weakness (usually sparing the face; however, when the face is involved it is less prominent). This is a result of the involvement of the pyramidal tract. Weakness that spares the face can mimic a cervical cord localization.

❏ Contralateral decreased position and vibration sense, as a result of the involvement of the medial lemniscus.

❏ Ipsilateral tongue weakness from the involvement of the hypoglossal nucleus (cranial nerve XII) and exiting fascicles (tongue deviates toward the side of the lesion).

4.2 Inferior medial pontine syndrome (Foville syndrome)

This pontine syndrome (Fig. 4.18) results from occlusion of the basilar perforators (paramedian branches).

The neurological symptoms associated with this syndrome include:

❏ Ipsilateral conjugate lateral gaze palsy from the involvement of the nucleus of cranial nerve six.

❏ Ipsilateral facial weakness. This is a result of the involvement of the facial colliculus.

❏ Contralateral hemibody weakness from the involvement of the corticospinal tract.

❏ Contralateral vibration/proprioception loss. This is from the involvement of the medial lemniscus.

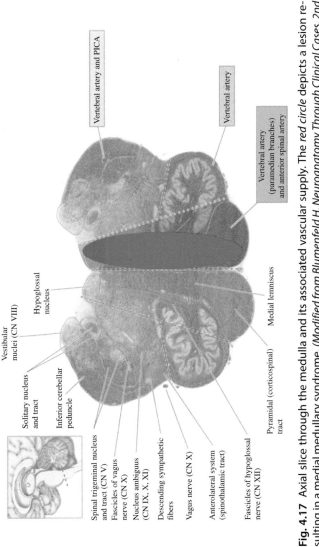

Fig. 4.17 Axial slice through the medulla and its associated vascular supply. The *red circle* depicts a lesion resulting in a medial medullary syndrome. (Modified from Blumenfeld H. *Neuroanatomy Through Clinical Cases*. 2nd ed. Oxford University Press; 2010, Copyright (2010) Oxford University Press.)

Vertebral artery and PICA

Vertebral artery

Vertebral artery (paramedian branches) and anterior spinal artery

Vestibular nuclei (CN VIII)

Hypoglossal nucleus

Solitary nucleus and tract

Inferior cerebellar peduncle

Medial lemniscus

Spinal trigeminal nucleus and tract (CN V)

Fascicles of vagus nerve (CN X)

Nucleus ambiguus (CN IX, X, XI)

Descending sympathetic fibers

Vagus nerve (CN X)

Anterolateral system (spinothalamic tract)

Fascicles of hypoglossal nerve (CN XII)

Pyramidal (corticospinal) tract

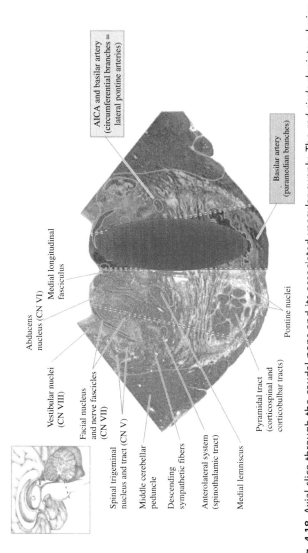

Fig. 4.18 Axial slice through the caudal pons and its associated vascular supply. The *red circle* depicts a lesion resulting in an inferior medial pontine syndrome (Foville syndrome). *(Modified from Blumenfeld H. Neuroanatomy Through Clinical Cases. 2nd ed. Oxford University Press; 2010, Copyright (2010) Oxford University Press.)*

Abducens
nucleus (CN VI)

Medial longitudinal
fasciculus

Vestibular nuclei
(CN VIII)

Facial nucleus
and nerve fascicles
(CN VII)

Spinal trigeminal
nucleus and tract (CN V)

Middle cerebellar
peduncle

Descending
sympathetic fibers

Anterolateral system
(spinothalamic tract)

Medial lemniscus

Pyramidal tract
(corticospinal and
corticobulbar tracts)

Pontine nuclei

AICA and basilar artery
(circumferential branches =
lateral pontine arteries)

Basilar artery
(paramedian branches)

4.3 Inferior lateral pontine syndrome (Marie-Foix syndrome)

This syndrome (Fig. 4.19) is caused by occlusion of the anterior inferior cerebellar artery (AICA).

The neurological symptoms associated with this syndrome include:

❏ Ipsilateral ataxia from the involvement of the middle cerebellar peduncle.
❏ Ipsilateral Horner's syndrome as the descending sympathetic chain runs through this area.
❏ Vertigo/hearing changes from involvement of the eighth cranial nerve nucleus or vestibular apparatus/cochlea (supplied by labyrinthine artery which branches from the AICA).
❏ Ipsilateral facial pain/temperature loss. Spinal trigeminal nucleus and tract courses through this area.
❏ Contralateral loss of the pain/temperature from spinothalamic tract involvement.
❏ Ipsilateral facial paralysis from the seventh fascicular involvement.

4.4 Medial mid-pontine syndrome

The neurological symptoms associated with this syndrome include (Fig. 4.20):

❏ Ipsilateral ataxia (from crossing cerebellar fibers).
❏ Contralateral hemibody weakness from the involvement of the corticospinal tract.
❏ Contralateral vibration/proprioception loss (medial lemniscus)—if lesion is large enough.

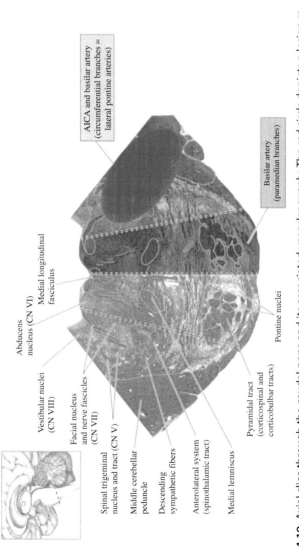

Fig. 4.19 Axial slice through the caudal pons and its associated vascular supply. The *red circle* depicts a lesion resulting in an inferior lateral pontine syndrome (Marie-Foix syndrome). *(Modified from Blumenfeld H. Neuroanatomy Through Clinical Cases. 2nd ed. Oxford University Press; 2010, Copyright (2010) Oxford University Press.)*

AICA and basilar artery (circumferential branches = lateral pontine arteries)

Basilar artery (paramedian branches)

Abducens nucleus (CN VI)

Medial longitudinal fasciculus

Vestibular nuclei (CN VIII)

Facial nucleus and nerve fascicles (CN VII)

Spinal trigeminal nucleus and tract (CN V)

Middle cerebellar peduncle

Descending sympathetic fibers

Anterolateral system (spinothalamic tract)

Medial lemniscus

Pyramidal tract (corticospinal and corticobulbar tracts)

Pontine nuclei

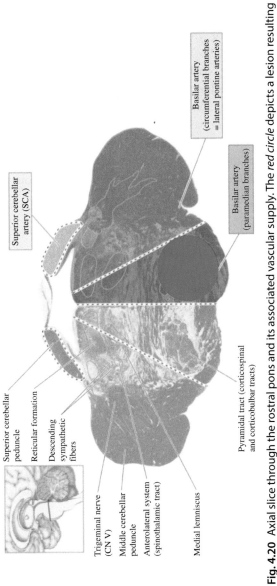

Fig. 4.20 Axial slice through the rostral pons and its associated vascular supply. The *red circle* depicts a lesion resulting in a medial mid-pontine syndrome. *(Modified from Blumenfeld H. Neuroanatomy Through Clinical Cases. 2nd ed. Oxford University Press; 2010, Copyright (2010) Oxford University Press.)*

Superior cerebellar peduncle

Reticular formation

Descending sympathetic fibers

Trigeminal nerve (CN V)

Middle cerebellar peduncle

Anterolateral system (spinothalamic tract)

Medial lemniscus

Superior cerebellar artery (SCA)

Basilar artery (circumferential branches = lateral pontine arteries)

Basilar artery (paramedian branches)

Pyramidal tract (corticospinal and corticobulbar tracts)

4.5 Lateral mid-pontine syndrome

The neurological symptoms associated with this syndrome include (Fig. 4.21):

❏ Ipsilateral ataxia from the involvement of the middle cerebellar peduncle.
❏ Ipsilateral facial numbness from the involvement of the fifth cranial nerve
❏ Ipsilateral paralysis of mastication from motor involvement of the fifth cranial nerve.
❏ Contralateral loss of the pain/temperature from spinothalamic tract involvement.

4.6 Midbrain peduncle (Weber syndrome)

The neurological symptoms associated with this syndrome include (Fig. 4.22):

❏ Ipsilateral third nerve palsy from the involvement of the fascicle of cranial nerve three.
❏ Contralateral hemibody weakness from the involvement of the cerebral peduncle.

4.7 Dorsomedial midbrain (Claude syndrome)

The neurological symptoms associated with this syndrome include (Fig. 4.23):

❏ Ipsilateral third nerve palsy from the involvement of the fascicle of cranial nerve 3.
❏ Contralateral (or ipsilateral) tremor and ataxia from the involvement of the red nucleus and cerebellothalamic fibers.

4.8 Paramedian midbrain (Benedikt syndrome)

Deficits include a combined Weber and Claude syndrome (Fig. 4.24):

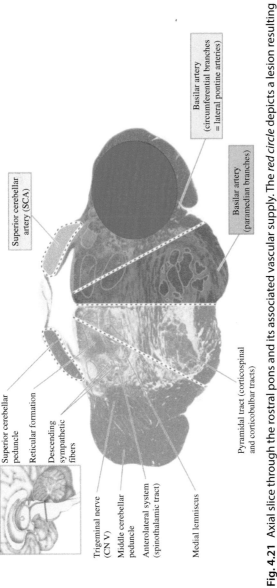

Fig. 4.21 Axial slice through the rostral pons and its associated vascular supply. The *red circle* depicts a lesion resulting in a lateral mid-pontine syndrome. *(Modified from Blumenfeld H. Neuroanatomy Through Clinical Cases. 2nd ed. Oxford University Press; 2010, Copyright (2010) Oxford University Press.)*

Superior cerebellar artery (SCA)

Basilar artery (circumferential branches = lateral pontine arteries)

Basilar artery (paramedian branches)

Superior cerebellar peduncle

Reticular formation

Descending sympathetic fibers

Trigeminal nerve (CN V)

Middle cerebellar peduncle

Anterolateral system (spinothalamic tract)

Medial lemniscus

Pyramidal tract (corticospinal and corticobulbar tracts)

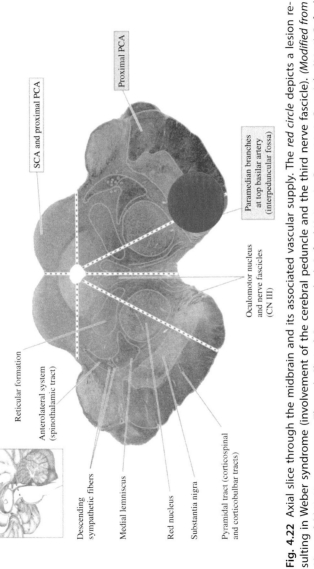

Fig. 4.22 Axial slice through the midbrain and its associated vascular supply. The *red circle* depicts a lesion resulting in Weber syndrome (involvement of the cerebral peduncle and the third nerve fascicle). *(Modified from Blumenfeld H. Neuroanatomy Through Clinical Cases. 2nd ed. Oxford University Press; 2010, Copyright (2010) Oxford University Press.)*

SCA and proximal PCA

Proximal PCA

Paramedian branches at top basilar artery (interpeduncular fossa)

Oculomotor nucleus and nerve fascicles (CN III)

Reticular formation

Anterolateral system (spinothalamic tract)

Descending sympathetic fibers

Medial lemniscus

Red nucleus

Substantia nigra

Pyramidal tract (corticospinal and corticobulbar tracts)

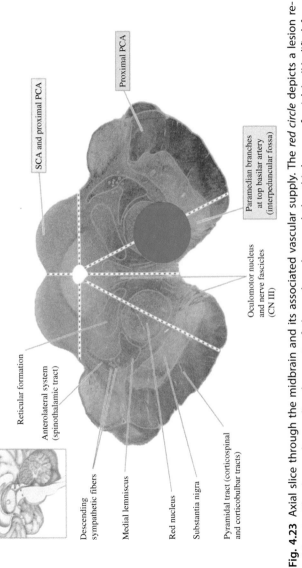

Fig. 4.23 Axial slice through the midbrain and its associated vascular supply. The *red circle* depicts a lesion resulting in Claude syndrome (involvement of the red nucleus and the third nerve fascicle). *(Modified from Blumenfeld H. Neuroanatomy Through Clinical Cases. 2nd ed. Oxford University Press; 2010, Copyright (2010) Oxford University Press.)*

Labels in figure:

- SCA and proximal PCA
- Proximal PCA
- Paramedian branches at top basilar artery (interpeduncular fossa)
- Oculomotor nucleus and nerve fascicles (CN III)
- Reticular formation
- Anterolateral system (spinothalamic tract)
- Descending sympathetic fibers
- Medial lemniscus
- Red nucleus
- Substantia nigra
- Pyramidal tract (corticospinal and corticobulbar tracts)

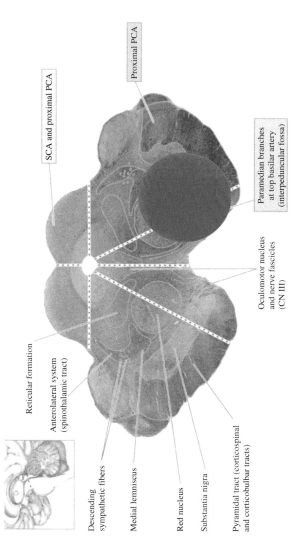

Fig. 4.24 Axial slice through the midbrain and its associated vascular supply. The *red circle* depicts a lesion resulting in Benedikt syndrome (involvement of the cerebral peduncle, red nucleus and the third nerve fascicle). *(Modified from Blumenfeld H. Neuroanatomy Through Clinical Cases. 2nd ed. Oxford University Press; 2010, Copyright (2010) Oxford University Press.)*

Reticular formation

Anterolateral system (spinothalamic tract)

SCA and proximal PCA

Proximal PCA

Paramedian branches at top basilar artery (interpeduncular fossa)

Oculomotor nucleus and nerve fascicles (CN III)

Descending sympathetic fibers

Medial lemniscus

Red nucleus

Substantia nigra

Pyramidal tract (corticospinal and corticobulbar tracts)

❏ Ipsilateral third nerve palsy from the involvement of the fascicle of cranial nerve 3.
❏ Contralateral hemibody weakness, tremor, and ataxia.
❏ May also have contralateral rigidity from the involvement of the substantia nigra.

5 SPINAL CORD SYNDROMES

The vascular supply of the spinal cord results from one anterior and two posterior spinal arteries. The **anterior spinal artery supplies the anterior two-thirds of the spinal cord, therefore supplying the corticospinal tract and spinothalamic tract. The posterior spinal artery supplies the dorsal columns.** The anterior spinal arteries are branches of the vertebral arteries with additional blood supply from radicular arteries of the thoracic and abdominal aorta (Fig. 4.25). The largest of these branches is the artery of Adamkiewicz (anywhere from T9 to T12) which supplies the anterior spinal artery. The primary watershed area for most people is in the midthoracic area. There are two main stroke syndromes in the spinal cord; the (i) anterior and (ii) posterior spinal cord syndrome.

5.1 Anterior spinal artery syndrome

The neurological symptoms associated with this syndrome include:
❏ Ipsilateral weakness below the level of ischemia/infarction.
❏ Contralateral pain/temperature loss contralateral to the level of ischemia/infarction.

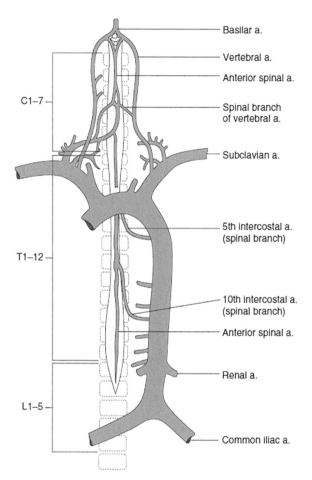

Fig. 4.25 Spinal cord vasculature. *(Reproduced with permission from Grotta J, et al. Stroke: Pathophysiology, Diagnosis, and Management. 6th ed. Canada: Elsevier, 2015, Copyright (2015) Elsevier Canada.)*

- Acute spinal shock resulting in lower extremity flaccid tone and hyporeflexia that is replaced in the next few days with upper motor neuron signs of spasticity and hyperreflexia.
- There may be associated autonomic symptoms such as hypotension, sexual dysfunction, and bowel/bladder dysfunction.

Note: Posterior column function is spared.

5.2 Posterior spinal artery syndrome

The neurological symptoms associated with this syndrome include:

- Ipsilateral hemisensory loss (proprioception, vibration, and touch) below the level of ischemia/infarction.
- There may be associated autonomic symptoms such as hypotension, sexual dysfunction, and bowel/bladder dysfunction.

6 THALAMIC SYNDROMES

The arterial supply to the thalamus comes from perforators off the PCA and posterior communicating artery, or from the anterior choroidal artery. The perforators supply discrete functional divisions of the thalamus resulting in many different clinical presentations involving deficits in sensorimotor function, cognition, vision, coordination, aphasia, level of consciousness, and sleep–wake cycle. Thalamic strokes occur either in isolation (often a result of small vessel disease) or in conjunction with other posterior (or anterior in the case of anterior choroidal artery) circulation syndromes. Thalamic strokes can also occur from venous occlusion involving the deep venous system.

There are many described thalamic syndromes in the literature resulting from occlusion of different small perforators, however, a description of each syndrome is beyond the scope of this book. Below we will review a list of symptoms that can occur in isolation or in combination, depending on the topographic involvement of the thalamus (medial, lateral, anterior, or posterior).

Thalamic strokes can result in:

❏ Hemisensory impairment (face/arm/leg)
❏ Central pain syndrome (Dejerine Roussy syndrome)
❏ Hemiataxia
❏ Anterograde memory loss (involvement of anterior portion of thalamus), apathy and neuropsychiatric disturbances
❏ Visual field defect: homonymous hemianopia, quadrantanopsia, or sectoranopia (wedge-shaped visual defect)
❏ Transcortical aphasia (with dominant hemisphere lesions)
❏ Decreased level of consciousness (especially if bilateral thalami involvement), behavioral changes
❏ Hyperkinestic movement disorders (myoclonus, athetosis or athetoid posture, action tremor)

Summary

In this chapter, we reviewed the many common and less common stroke syndromes. This chapter may be a useful resource that you frequently come back to review, especially when faced with an uncommon stroke presentation. Understanding cerebral and spinal cord anatomy will help you apply your knowledge more readily in the clinical setting.

Thinking about the lesion's localization can enhance your appreciation of etiology, further guide imaging and other investigations, and direct treatment.

Further reading

1. Blumenfeld H. *Neuroanatomy Through Clinical Cases*. 2nd ed. Oxford University Press; 2010.
2. Caplan L. *Caplan's Stroke. A Clinical Approach*. 4th ed. Boston: Elsevier Canada; 2009.
3. Felten D, Maida M, Netter F, O'Banion M. *Netter's Atlas of Neuroscience*. 3rd ed. Canada: Elsevier; 2015.
4. Grotta J, et al. *Stroke: Pathophysiology, Diagnosis, and Management*. 6th ed. Canada: Elsevier; 2015.
5. Mandell J. *Core Radiology*. Cambridge University Press; 2013.
6. Mattle HP, et al. Basilar artery occlusion. *Lancet Neurol*. 2011;10(11):1002–1014.
7. Gates P. The rule of 4 of the brainstem: a simplified method for understanding brainstem anatomy and brainstem vascular syndromes for the non-neurologist. *Intern Med J*. 2005;35:263–266.

CHAPTER 5

Stroke imaging: Noncontrast head CT

The next set of imaging chapters will provide you with an organized approach to ordering and interpreting acute stroke imaging studies. To best assess a patient presenting with acute stroke symptoms, we ideally want imaging of the brain (neuroimaging) and imaging of the vessels (vascular imaging).

The goals of acute stroke imaging are threefold:

(1) Diagnosis—to help establish a rapid and accurate diagnosis of the type of stroke and the vascular lesion, and exclude mimics.

(2) Prognosis—to help predict outcome in terms of disability, risk of deterioration/complications/mortality, and risk of stroke recurrence.

(3) Treatment decision-making—to identify patients who would be candidates for thrombolysis, endovascular therapy, anticoagulation, or antiplatelet therapy. In addition to patient selection for acute treatments, imaging can also serve as a triage tool to help identify low-risk patients who can be discharged and high-risk patients who may require ICU admission.

In this chapter, we will specifically review an approach to interpretation of stroke imaging with a focus on noncontrast head CT: how to identify hemorrhage, hyperdense vessel signs, and signs of acute ischemia/infarction including the ASPECTS scoring system.

The Code Stroke Handbook   © 2020 Elsevier Inc. All rights reserved.
https://doi.org/10.1016/B978-0-12-820522-8.00005-3

> ## A multimodal CT acute stroke imaging protocol consists of
>
> 1. Noncontrast head CT
> 2. Multiphase contrast CT angiogram (CTA), from the aortic arch to vertex
> 3. Contrast CT brain perfusion study (CTP)

For years stroke imaging has been limited to a noncontrast head CT scan and a carotid Doppler ultrasound. The advent of advanced CT stroke imaging protocols now at many institutions (CTA and CTP) or MR imaging protocols (MRI, MRA, and MR perfusion) has revolutionized the field, improving stroke diagnosis and patient selection for acute reperfusion therapies. Current practice guidelines recommend urgent neurovascular imaging preferably in the form of head CT and CTA of the head and neck arteries. CTA can be completed in a couple of minutes and is the most efficient and sensitive diagnostic study for a complete assessment of the extracranial and intracranial circulation. In contrast, carotid ultrasound does not assess the intracranial vessels, the extracranial posterior circulation, or the aortic arch, and can miss many important etiologies including cervicocephalic artery dissections. A CT venogram can be requested if there is concern about cerebral venous sinus thrombosis.

What if a patient has acute or chronic kidney disease?

In general, iodine contrast dye has been relatively contraindicated in patients with a creatinine clearance < 30 mL/min. However, many recent studies have provided reassuring data indicating that the risk of contrast-induced nephropathy is quite low. According to a large study ($n = 21{,}346$) by McDonald et al.[1] the incidence of new cases of dialysis following contrast administration was less than 1%, and contrast administration was not associated with increased risk of acute kidney injury, dialysis, or death (even among patients with preexisting renal disease, diabetes, and other comorbidities). Therefore, in an emergency situation, when faced with a patient who is in the midst of a disabling acute stroke and may be eligible for treatment with tPA or endovascular therapy, most stroke specialists would agree that the brain takes priority ("*neurons over nephrons*"). In other words, if the results from a contrast $CTA \pm CTP$ study are likely to add value or change patient management, it is reasonable to go ahead and obtain a contrast study, and ideally in discussion with the patient (if possible) and family. Intravenous fluids can be administered after the scan to help eliminate the contrast dye. As well, iodine contrast can be dialyzed if the patient is already on intermittent dialysis. Nephrology may be consulted if needed. Given that time is of the essence in acute stroke management, it is not recommended to delay imaging and treatment while awaiting a creatinine result from the laboratory.

What if the patient has a known iodine contrast allergy?

For reactions such as hives, a common treatment regimen is hydrocortisone 200 mg IV and diphenhydramine 50-mg IV administered before, during or after the contrast CT scan to mitigate potential reactions. For patients with a past history of life-threatening reactions (anaphylaxis), an iodine contrast dye is best avoided, and instead, vascular imaging can be obtained by MR angiography or ultrasound (carotid Doppler and transcranial Doppler), where available.

Before we discuss code stroke imaging further, knowledge of the relevant neuroanatomy and vascular anatomy is important. Below we demonstrate anatomical structures on different slices of a normal noncontrast head CT (Figs. 5.1 and 5.2). <u>On a noncontrast head CT, the cerebrospinal fluid appears black; bone (and other calcifications) appears white</u>.

Standard nomenclature for describing lesions on CT or MRI is as follows:

On <u>CT</u> scan a lesion is referred to as hypo/
<u>hyperdense</u>.

On <u>MRI</u> scans it is referred to as hypo/
hyper<u>intense</u>.

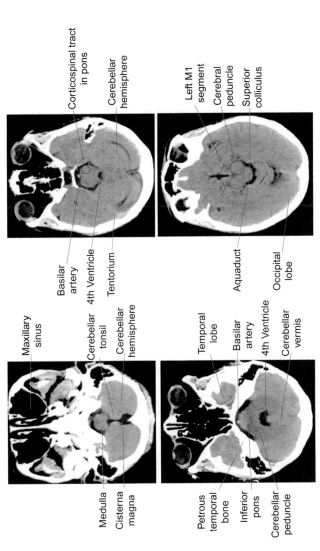

Fig. 5.1 Different slices of an axial noncontrast head CT with important structures labeled.

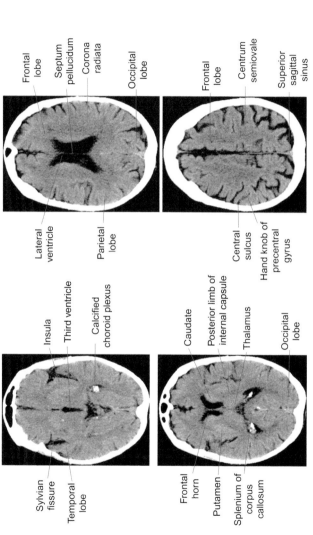

Fig. 5.2 Different slices of an axial noncontrast head CT with important structures labeled.

1 Approach to interpreting the acute noncontrast head CT

The noncontrast head CT is an extension of your history and neurological examination. Your history and NIHSS exam will guide where to focus your attention to pick up abnormalities on the noncontrast head CT.

The noncontrast CT scan can appear normal in the acute stroke setting (Fig. 5.3). Early acute ischemic changes on CT are often subtle and can be difficult to detect, and some infarcts are too small to be visible by CT.

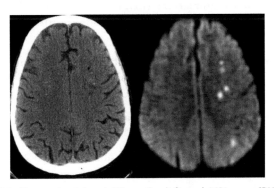

Fig. 5.3 Noncontrast head CT on the left and MRI scan (DWI sequence) on the right of the same patient at 4 h from symptom onset. The right DWI MRI sequence reveals tiny hyperintensities in the left hemisphere consistent with acute ischemic lesions that cannot be readily identified on the noncontrast CT head.

Interpretation of a noncontrast head CT in the acute stroke setting takes practice and should be done systematically every time. Below is a general four-step approach. It does not, however, replace a radiologist's interpretation.

> ### Four-step approach to reading a noncontrast head CT for acute stroke assessment
>
> **(1)** First look for the presence/absence of hemorrhage (intracerebral, subarachnoid, or subdural).
>   - Acute blood is hyperdense (bright)
>   - Subacute blood is isodense (similar density to brain parenchyma)
>   - Chronic blood is hypodense (darker than the brain)
>
> **(2)** Look for the presence/absence of any hyperdense vessel signs suggestive of an acute clot in a major artery (i.e., MCA sign, ACA, PCA, basilar) or vein (dural venous thrombosis or deep vein thrombosis).
>
> **(3)** Identify the presence/absence and extent of any early acute ischemic changes, which can be rated on the ASPECTS scale.
>
> **(4)** Exclude *other* structural brain pathology.

First look for any areas of abnormal hyperdensity (i.e., bright white on CT) that could represent acute or recent hemorrhage. Note that calcium and protein will also appear hyperdense on CT (i.e., the basal ganglia often shows bilateral calcifications in older individuals) although it looks as white as the skull bone and should not be confused with hemorrhage which is not quite as bright white. Look for subacute hemorrhage too. Small areas of subarachnoid hemorrhage or thin subdural hematomas can be subtle and easy to miss.

If the CT scan shows acute hemorrhage, then the patient does not qualify for intravenous tPA (absolute contraindication). We obtain a CTA to look for a potential underlying structural lesion (such as aneurysm, arteriovenous malformation, dural arteriovenous-fistula, or neoplasm) and to assess for the presence of a spot sign (will discuss this sign in the chapter on CTA).

Important radiographic components of an acute intracerebral (intraparenchymal) hemorrhage (ICH) to describe include:

❏ Location (infratentorial, deep subcortical, lobar)
❏ Volume in cm^3 (we will go through an example of how to calculate hematoma volume)
❏ Mass effect
❏ Intraventricular extension
❏ Hydrocephalus
❏ Imaging findings to suggest a secondary cause

Below we will review a few clinical vignettes with accompanying noncontrast CT scans.

A 78-year-old woman with chronic hypertension presents 2 h after the onset of acute confusion and right hemiparesis (face/ arm/leg). An urgent noncontrast CT scan was completed and is shown below Fig. 5.4.

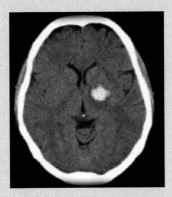

Fig. 5.4 CT scan reveals a small acute deep intracerebral hemorrhage in the region of the left globus pallidus, internal capsule, and part of the thalamus with a minimal amount of surrounding vasogenic edema and no midline shift.

A 32-year-old woman with a remote history of a deep vein thrombosis presents with headache and difficulty reading the left side of the newspaper. An urgent CT head is completed and shown below Fig. 5.5.

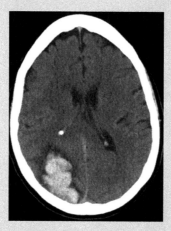

Fig. 5.5 CT scan reveals an acute lobar intracerebral hemorrhage located in the right posterior temporal-occipital region with mass effect and surrounding vasogenic edema.

On further imaging with CT venogram, she is found to have thrombosis of the superior sagittal sinus and right transverse sinus with resulting intraparenchymal hemorrhage.

How to calculate hematoma size

You can estimate the volume of a hematoma by using the $(A \times B \times C)/2$ *formula*, which is important as it is a predictor of morbidity and mortality.

In the formula, A stands for the greatest hematoma diameter in the axial plane (in cm), B is the hematoma diameter perpendicular to A (in cm), and C is the number of CT slices on which the hematoma is visible multiplied by the slice thickness (usually 0.5 cm). If the measurements are in centimeters, then the volume will be calculated in cubic centimeters (cm^3 or mL).

Let us go through an example Fig. 5.6:

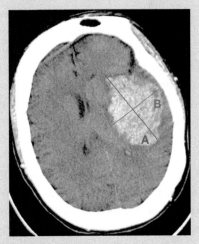

Fig. 5.6 Calculating hematoma size.

This is a noncontrast head CT scan of a large acute intraparenchymal hematoma in the left lentiform nucleus extending to the adjacent frontal and temporal lobe, with associated rightward midline shift. In this case, **A** measures 6.9 cm and **B** measures 5.1 cm. The hematoma is visible on eight slices and the slice thickness is 0.5 cm (**C** = 4). Therefore, the hematoma volume is $(6.9 \times 5.1 \times 4)/2 = 70\,\text{cm}^3$.

Depending on local practice ICH can be managed by stroke specialists. Neurosurgery is often consulted when there is intraventricular extension, midline shift from mass effect, cerebellar hemorrhage, or hydrocephalus. Hemorrhage isolated to the subarachnoid space, subdural or epidural space is primarily managed by neurosurgery.

The etiology of ICH is beyond the focus of this book, however, we will briefly discuss an approach as it will help with interpreting neuroimaging. ICH is often divided into *primary* and *secondary*, of which hypertension and cerebral amyloid angiopathy are the etiologies for primary ICH. Hypertension is a risk factor for small vessel disease. Deep hemorrhages from rupture of tiny blood vessels (i.e., located in the basal ganglia, thalamus, pons, or cerebellum) are typically associated with small vessel disease (with chronic hypertension as the main culprit). Other radiographic signs of small vessel disease are often seen including chronic white matter microangiopathic changes and microhemorrhages (seen on GRE sequence of MRI).

Lobar ICH refers to hemorrhages that are located close to the surface of the brain (superficial) within the frontal, temporal, parietal or occipital lobes. Such hemorrhages are typically associated with cerebral amyloid angiopathy in older patients. In young patients, search for an underlying lesion or secondary cause.

ICH prognostic scales have been developed to predict clinical outcomes. One scale, the ICH Score by Hemphill et al.[2] is shown below. The total score is the summation of all 5 components and a maximum score is 6. The higher the cumulative score the higher the 30-day mortality (columns 3 and 4).

ICH score			
Component	Points	Total ICH score	30-day mortality (%)
Glascow coma scale		0	0–10
3–4	2		
5–12	1		
13–15	0		
Age (years)		1	7–13
≥80	1		
<80	0		
ICH volume (mL)		2	30–44
≥30	1		
<30	0		
Presence of intraventricular hemorrhage		3	56–78
Yes	1		
No	0		
Infratentorial origin of ICH		4	70–100
Yes	1		
No	0		
Total ICH score	/6	5–6	100

Hemphill JC, Bonovich DC, Besmertis L, Manley GT, Johnston SC. The ICH score: a simple, reliable grading scale for intracerebral hemorrhage. *Stroke* 2001;32(4):891–897.

Remember that a primary ischemic stroke can undergo secondary hemorrhagic transformation (Fig. 5.7), so CT evidence of hemorrhage does not automatically rule out an initial infarction. The presence of surrounding hypodensity in a vascular territory or a vascular occlusion on CT angiogram may help in diagnosing hemorrhagic transformation of an infarct.

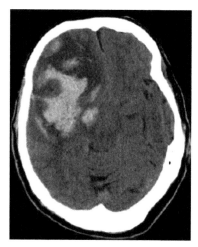

Fig. 5.7 Right middle cerebral artery infarct with secondary hemorrhagic transformation and resultant midline shift.

2 Hyperdense vessel signs

A hyperdense vessel sign is direct visualization of an acute thrombus in an intracranial artery. In the middle cerebral artery, a hyperdense vessel can be seen in the proximal segment (M1) or distal M2 or M3 branches, i.e., Sylvian dot sign signifying distal MCA branch occlusion in the Sylvian fissure. An M1 or proximal M2 occlusion is important to identify as it is a potential target for urgent endovascular therapy. The location and length of the clot have prognostic value and correlate with the likelihood of recanalization and treatment outcomes.

In many, but not all, large vessel occlusions, there will be a hyperdense vessel sign visible on noncontrast head CT prior to the CT angiogram. This is a result of the composition of the clot, as more dense clots are seen on CT which are red blood cell-rich, compared to fibrin-rich clots which are less dense and less often seen on noncontrast CT.

It is helpful when trying to identify a hyperdense vessel, to compare to the contralateral (normal) side. If the patient was recently administered IV contrast (i.e., underwent a recent CT angiogram or after cardiac catheterization), then the vessels will all look hyperdense.

We will review a few examples of hyperdense MCA signs (depicted by the red arrow) seen on noncontrast CT head (Fig. 5.8).

In addition to the MCA hyperdense vessel sign, direct visualization of clot can also be seen in the basilar artery—a hyperdense basilar sign. Because of the limitations of CT for the posterior fossa (limited spatial resolution and streak artifact from surrounding bone structures), a hyperdense basilar sign can be overcalled, and unfortunately, undercalled. A good review of the basilar should be part of your approach to reading the noncontrast head CT, especially if the patient is presenting with posterior circulation stroke symptoms. We review two examples of a hyperdense basilar artery seen on noncontrast head CT (Fig. 5.9). Again, always pursue CTA for definitive diagnosis of any potential vascular occlusion.

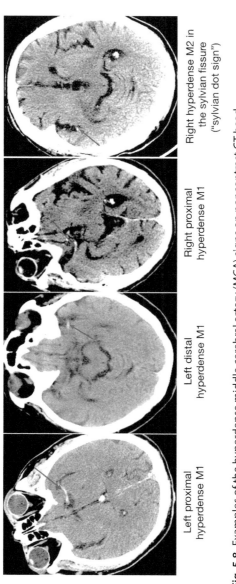

Fig. 5.8 Examples of the hyperdense middle cerebral artery (MCA) signs on noncontrast CT head.

Left proximal hyperdense M1

Left distal hyperdense M1

Right proximal hyperdense M1

Right hyperdense M2 in the sylvian fissure ("sylvian dot sign")

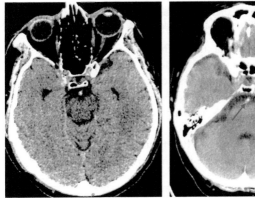

Fig. 5.9 Noncontrast head CT with a *red arrow* labeling the hyperdense basilar artery.

3 Acute ischemic changes on CT head (ASPECTS score)

Early signs of ischemia can be identified by looking for a loss of gray-white matter differentiation and/or gyral effacement. Over time you will learn to train your eye to detect the subtle early changes. A helpful tip is to look at the "normal" side to identify asymmetry. Look also for areas of hypodensity, which develop later and correlate with infarction of tissue.

The ASPECTS scoring system is a validated standardized rating system developed by the Calgary Stroke Program to quantify the extent of early ischemic changes and can help select potential candidates for tPA and endovascular therapy (more on its application for thrombolytic/endovascular therapy in the treatment chapters). It can only be used for strokes that affect the internal carotid artery or middle cerebral artery and does not apply to the anterior cerebral artery or posterior circulation.

To maximize the detection of loss of gray-white differentiation, you may adjust your CT "window settings." We recommend a CT window width of 40 and a window level of 40.

Aspects scoring system

One point is subtracted from 10 for any evidence of early ischemic change in each of the defined regions below. An important point to know is that only areas of acute ischemia are scored. A total of six points is assigned to different MCA segments (these do not correspond to the distal MCA branches) and 4 points to deep structures. A total score of 10 reflects a normal CT scan with no evidence of acute ischemic change.

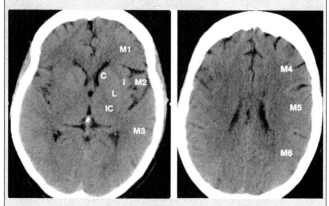

Fig. 5.10 The 10 defined regions of the ASPECTS scoring system labeled on noncontrast head CT scans; created by the authors. (1) C, Caudate; (2) IC, posterior internal capsule (note: only the genu and posterior limb are scored); (3) I, insular cortex; (4) L, lentiform nucleus; (5) M1, anterior MCA cortex; (6) M2, MCA cortex lateral to the insular ribbon; (7) M3, posterior MCA cortex; (8) M4, anterior MCA territory at the level of the lateral ventricle; (9) M5, lateral MCA territory at the level of the lateral ventricle; (10) M6, posterior MCA territory at the level of the lateral ventricle.

We will review the standardized scoring system below Fig. 5.10.

Let us review examples of loss of gray-white differentiation (area in red circle) (Fig. 5.11).

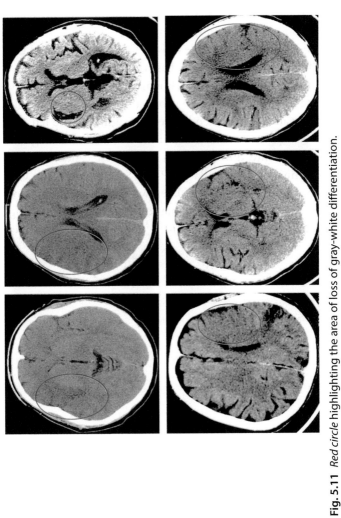

Fig. 5.11 *Red circle* highlighting the area of loss of gray-white differentiation.

As mentioned above, the ASPECTS scoring system is designed for ICA and MCA strokes. There is no universally accepted scoring system for the posterior circulation, however, one that can be used is the posterior circulation ASPECTS (pc-ASPECTS). A review of this scale, however, is beyond the scope of this handbook.

Fig. 5.12 is an example of ischemic changes seen in the posterior circulation from a basilar thrombus.

Fig. 5.13 is an example showing the evolution of early acute ischemic changes to subacute changes on noncontrast head CT. In the code stroke imaging on the left, we see two different axial slices of the head CT showing loss of gray-white differentiation in the left caudate, lentiform nucleus and insula (ASPECTS score of 7). The CT scan on the right, 3 days later we see the evolution of the left MCA stroke with acute hyperdensity signifying hemorrhagic transformation.

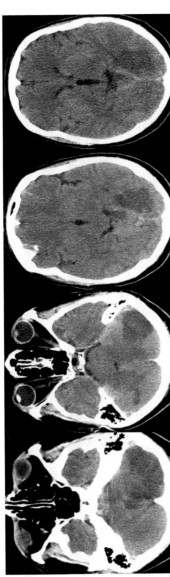

Fig. 5.12 Noncontrast head CT showing hypodensities in the bilateral cerebellum (left greater than right) associated with mass effect and partial effacement of the fourth ventricle, and left cerebellar tonsillar herniation. As well as there is hypodensity in the left tempo–occipital lobe. On the patient's CT angiogram (not shown here) there is focal occlusion of the left vertebral artery and a resultant filling defect in the basilar artery accounting for the above findings. The patient was taken for urgent endovascular therapy.

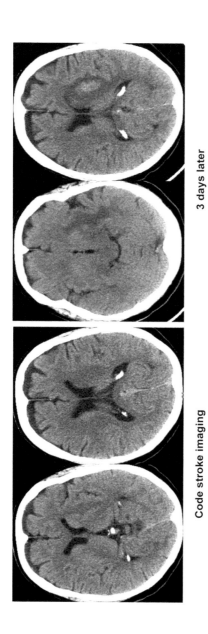

Code stroke imaging

3 days later

Fig. 5.13 Evolution of a left MCA stroke at the time of code stroke (images on left) and 3 days later post-EVT (images on right) with the new acute hemorrhagic transformation (hyperdensity within stroke).

4 Identifying other structural lesions

As mentioned in the stroke mimics section in Chapter 2, there are many stroke mimics that may be identified by CT. Intracranial pathology such as neoplasm (primary or metastatic), cytotoxic edema, demyelinating lesions, or certain infections (i.e., brain abscess and herpes simplex viral encephalitis) can mimic stroke. Neoplastic and infectious lesions can break down the blood–brain barrier, increasing the probability of detection when contrast is used.

We will review some other pathologies that may be picked up on acute stroke imaging.

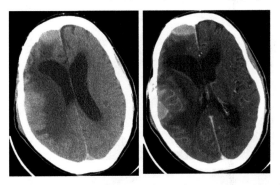

Fig. 5.14 Noncontrast head CT (left) and postcontrast head CT (right) revealing multiple meningiomas in the right hemisphere with associated cytotoxic edema.

In Fig. 5.14 we see multiple extra-axial lesions in the right hemisphere (on noncontrast and postcontrast CT scans) consistent with meningiomas with associated significant right hemisphere cytotoxic edema.

Fig. 5.15 shows examples of "other intracranial pathology" presenting as stroke mimics with sudden onset of neurological symptoms.

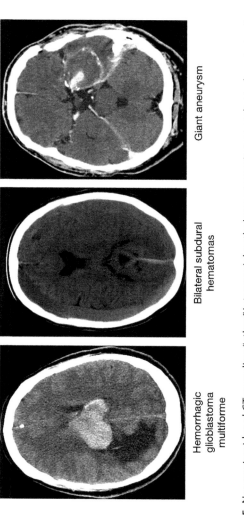

Fig. 5.15 Noncontrast head CT revealing "other" intracranial pathology presenting as code stroke mimics. From left to right; hemorrhagic glioblastoma multiforme, bilateral acute on chronic subdural hematomas, and giant internal carotid artery aneurysm.

Hemorrhagic glioblastoma multiforme

Bilateral subdural hematomas

Giant aneurysm

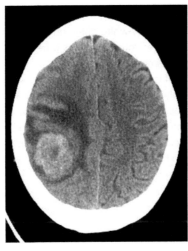

Fig. 5.16 Noncontrast head CT revealing a right frontoparietal mass with surrounding edema.

A code stroke activated for a 62-year-old woman with left-sided weakness, numbness, and left visual extinction.

Fig. 5.16 is her noncontrast head CT scan showing a right frontoparietal mass lesion with surrounding edema. The worsening edema is the likely culprit for her acute neurological symptoms.

Summary
A noncontrast head CT is used to identify areas of hyperdensity signifying an acute hemorrhage, identify a hyperdense vessel in the anterior or posterior circulation, identify the extent of acute ischemia/infarction which can be guided by the ASPECTS scale, identify subacute and chronic infarcts and white matter disease, and to exclude *other* structural lesions. Do not become discouraged if you find it difficult to assess

for subtle loss of gray-white differentiation on noncontrast CT head early on in your training as it becomes easier with practice and experience.

A couple of important points to remember: (i) to administer thrombolytics, all that is needed is a noncontrast head CT—to exclude hemorrhage and assess for eligibility, (ii) brain imaging is the only way to know for sure if an acute stroke is ischemic or hemorrhagic. In the next chapter, we will review the next imaging modality in the code stroke—the CT angiogram.

References and Further Reading

1. McDonald RJ, McDonald JS, Carter RE, et al. Intravenous contrast material exposure is not an independent risk factor for dialysis or mortality. *Radiology*. 2014;273:714–725.
2. Hemphill JC, Bonovich DC, Besmertis L, Manley GT, Johnston SC. The ICH score: a simple, reliable grading scale for intracerebral hemorrhage. *Stroke*. 2001;32(4):891–897.
3. ASPECT Score in Acute Stroke. University of Calgary http://aspectsinstroke.com/.
4. Brinjikji W, Krings T. *Imaging in Neurovascular Disease. A Case-Based Approach*. 1st ed. Thieme Publishers; 2020.
5. Warwick Pexman JH, Barber P, Hill M, et al. Use of the Alberta stroke program early CT score (ASPECTS) for assessing CT scans in patients with acute stroke. *Am J Neuroradiol*. 2001;22(8):1534–1542.

CHAPTER 6

Stroke imaging: CT angiography

In this chapter, we provide a general introduction to the use and interpretation of CT angiography for patients with acute ischemic stroke or TIA.
- ❏ Identifying the presence of an intracranial arterial occlusion with a focus on occlusions amenable to EVT.
- ❏ Identifying extracranial artery stenosis or dissection.
- ❏ Identifying cerebral venous sinus thrombosis.
This chapter also briefly discusses the use of CTA for patients presenting with acute intracerebral hemorrhage.

CT angiography (CTA) for acute stroke evaluation is best obtained right after the noncontrast head CT scan. It should be ordered as a "CTA from the aortic arch to vertex," as a CTA of the head only (i.e., "circle of Willis" scan) misses the extracranial vessels and a CTA of the neck only misses the intracranial circulation. CTA is more sensitive for detecting intra/extracranial stenosis or occlusion than MR angiography.

CTA in the acute stroke setting has three main goals

(1) **To identify the presence or absence of an intracranial occlusion (arterial or venous) that accounts for the clinical signs and symptoms, with a specific focus on identifying occlusions of the major arteries that may be amenable to EVT,** i.e., the proximal MCA (M1 segment or proximal M2 branches), proximal ACA, proximal PCA, extracranial or intracranial carotid, or basilar artery. In this way, the results of CTA can provide essential information about the stroke diagnosis and prognosis can help guide acute treatment decision-making for tPA and can identify potential candidates for EVT.

(2) **To identify significant stenosis/atherosclerosis or dissection at the aortic arch, common carotid artery, internal carotid artery, vertebral arteries, or intracranial arteries.** Such results are important for determining the most likely etiology when evaluating a patient with ischemic stroke or TIA and for guiding the most appropriate treatments for secondary stroke prevention.

(3) **For patients with acute intracerebral hemorrhage, to evaluate for intracranial aneurysm, vascular malformations, or other secondary causes for the hemorrhage. The presence or absence of a CTA "spot sign" can have prognostic value for the risk of early ICH expansion.**

1 Intracranial vessel occlusions

We will go through a few examples of M1 occlusions seen on CTA (Fig. 6.1). At most centers, CTA involves both source images (these are the thinner cuts) and the thick

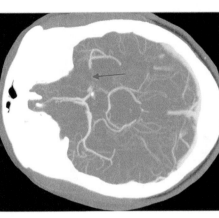

Left M1 occlusion (red arrow) seen on axial or coronal CT angiogram.

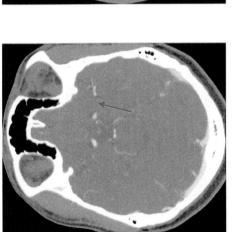

Thick axial CTA showing left M1 occlusion (in the same patient as left)

Left M1 occlusion over a 1.2 cm segment

Fig. 6.1 M1 occlusions (*red arrow*) seen on axial or coronal CT angiogram.

(Continued)

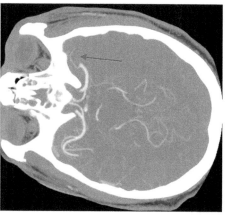

Right M1 occlusion seen on coronal CTA

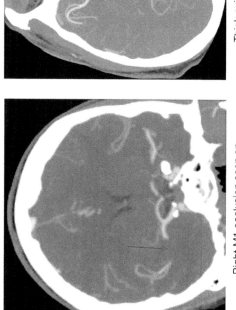

Thick axial CTA showing left distal M1 occlusion

Fig. 6.1, Cont'd

axial/coronal/sagittal MIP images. The axial MIP images are often very good at identifying a proximal MCA (M1) occlusion.

Here are examples of basilar occlusions seen on CTA (Figs. 6.2 and 6.3).

Below is a scroll-through of a CT angiogram showing basilar artery tapering to complete occlusion (an ominous sign) (Fig. 6.4).

Cerebral venous sinus thrombosis

A less frequent cause of ischemic stroke and hemorrhage is cerebral venous sinus thrombosis (CVST), and depending on the demographics of the patient and their presenting symptoms, you may have a higher index of clinical suspicion. Patients with inherited thrombophilias, hypercoagulable state, pregnancy/post-partum, birth control, trauma, and less commonly infection or systemic inflammatory diseases are at higher risk. Their clinical presentation does not localize to an arterial supply and often headache is an accompanying and predominant symptom. Patients are often young and can present with new persistent headaches, stroke symptoms, seizures, or raised intracranial pressure with papilledema. Recognition of CVST is important because the usual treatment is immediate anticoagulation. The noncontrast head CT is often deceptively normal and is insufficient to rule out this diagnosis; if CVST is suspected, a post-contrast head CT and ideally a CT venogram (CTV) is necessary.

There are radiographic signs on noncontrast and post-contrast head CT for CVST (Fig. 6.5):

❏ Hyperdensity in the corresponding occluded sinus
❏ Infarction, edema, or hemorrhage that crosses arterial boundaries or in close proximity to a venous sinus

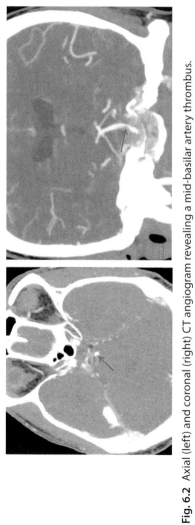

Fig. 6.2 Axial (left) and coronal (right) CT angiogram revealing a mid-basilar artery thrombus.

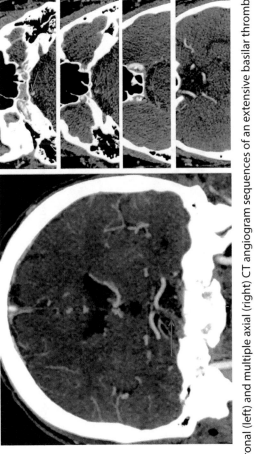

Fig. 6.3 Coronal (left) and multiple axial (right) CT angiogram sequences of an extensive basilar thrombus.

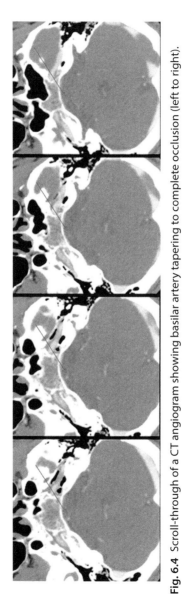

Fig. 6.4 Scroll-through of a CT angiogram showing basilar artery tapering to complete occlusion (left to right).

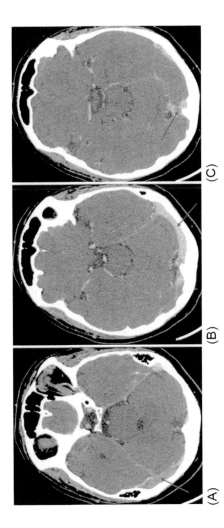

Fig. 6.5 Postcontrast head CT with *red arrows* showing: (A) a filling defect in the right transverse sinus (consistent with a venous thrombus), (B) a normal filling left transverse sinus, as a comparison, and (C) a filling defect in the torcula.

❑ Bilateral parenchymal involvement
❑ The delta sign on noncontrast head CT—results from thrombus in the posterior portion of the superior sagittal sinus
❑ The empty delta sign on postcontrast scan—thrombus seen in the superior sagittal sinus

2 Identifying extracranial carotid stenosis or dissection

CTA from the aortic arch to vertex not only helps to identify intracranial vessel occlusions as a target for EVT in acute stroke management, but it also helps to determine the cause of the stroke, as well as the ease of access for the EVT procedure itself. Carotid atherosclerosis (causing mild, moderate, or severe stenosis), extracranial arterial dissection, and carotid webs are possible etiologies of stroke that can be detected by CTA. Atherosclerotic plaque morphology (e.g. ulceration) can help with risk stratification.

Carotid atherosclerotic disease:

About 25% of all ischemic strokes can be attributed to large vessel atherosclerosis and approximately 7%–10% overall is due to carotid atherosclerosis. Patients with anterior circulation ischemic stroke or TIA and ipsilateral 50%–99% carotid stenosis have a high early risk of stroke recurrence.

According to one systematic review, the early risk of stroke recurrence in the context of symptomatic carotid disease can be as high as 26% within 2 weeks.[1]

Early treatment of symptomatic carotid disease with surgery (endarterectomy) or stenting is highly effective for reducing stroke risk and should ideally be performed as soon as possible within 2 weeks of the ischemic event, requiring urgent referral to an experienced carotid surgeon for consultation. In contrast, an incidental finding of <u>asymptomatic</u> carotid artery stenosis is generally treated medically, not surgically.

Fig. 6.6 is an example of significant left internal carotid artery atherosclerosis in a patient presenting with transient right hand weakness.

Extracranial vertebral artery atherosclerosis and aortic arch atheroma are also important causes of acute ischemic stroke that can be identified on CTA imaging. Although atherosclerosis in these locations is not usually treated with stenting or surgery, aggressive management of vascular risk factors and antiplatelet therapy is recommended.

Extracranial carotid and vertebral artery dissection:

Extracranial cervicocephalic artery dissection accounts for 2.5% of all strokes and is a common cause of stroke in the young. It accounts for up to 20% of strokes in patients < 45-years old. Arterial dissection occurs because of a tear in the intima resulting in an intramural hematoma. This, in turn, causes the release of endothelins, activation of platelets and the coagulation cascade, and may lead to luminal thrombus with distal embolization or vessel occlusion. Patients with arterial dissection often have a preceding history of head/neck trauma, neck manipulation, prolonged neck hyperextension, excessive coughing or vomiting prior to their presentation. However, arterial dissection can also occur spontaneously without an apparent trigger in otherwise healthy patients, or in patients with predisposing conditions such as Marfan syndrome, Ehlers Danlos syndrome, or fibromuscular dysplasia (to name a few).

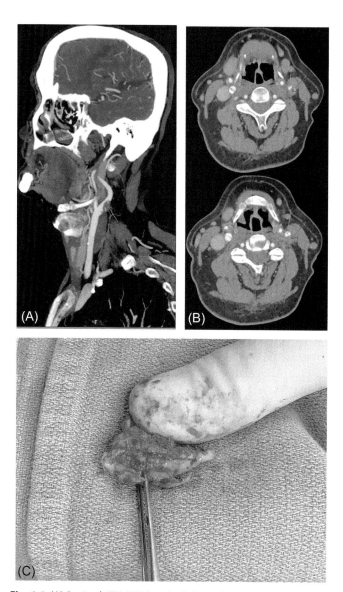

Fig. 6.6 (A) Sagittal CTA MIP (on the left) and (B) two axial thin slices (on right) through the significant plaque seen just above the left carotid bifurcation in the internal carotid artery (depicted by *red arrows*) with a residual lumen of 1.8 mm *(blue arrow)*, or about 50% stenosis. In (C) we see an example of atherosclerotic plaque removed by carotid endarterectomy. Photo courtesy of Dr. Ahmed Kayssi.

Patients will often complain of preceding head or neck pain prior to their ischemic stroke symptoms. With extracranial carotid dissection patients may have an ipsilateral Horner syndrome (third-order sympathetic fibers travel within the carotid sheath), monocular vision loss (the ICA supplies the ophthalmic artery), and other cranial nerve palsies (IX, X, XI, or XII because of their proximity to the carotid sheath).

Extracranial carotid or vertebral artery dissection is not a contraindication to thrombolysis. However, if a dissection extends intracranially, there is a small risk of subarachnoid hemorrhage if the tear extends through the adventitia. Although arterial dissection is also not a contraindication to EVT, access during the procedure may be more difficult.

There are certain clues to the diagnosis of extracranial arterial dissection on CTA. However, other than the visualization of an intimal flap, none are specific for dissection, and ultimately the patient history and age are important factors in the clinical suspicion for this etiology. Visualizing methemoglobin within the vessel wall on MRI may help to confirm the diagnosis.

CTA imaging findings in extracranial arterial dissection include:

❑ Intimal flap (Fig. 6.7)
❑ Tapered, "flame-shaped" occlusion
❑ "String sign"—a long, narrow, irregular column of contrast material that begins 2–3 cm distal to the carotid bulb extending to the base of the skull or starting at the V3 segment of the vertebral artery
❑ Pseudoaneurysm formation

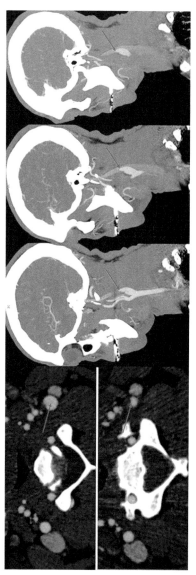

Fig. 6.7 Axial CTA thin slices on the left show an intimal flap *(red arrow)* and a reduction in lumen size of the left internal carotid artery. On the sagittal CTA MIP sequences, we see a tapered, "flame–" shaped occlusion *(red arrow)*.

In extracranial carotid dissection, the imaging abnormalities usually start 2–3 cm beyond the carotid bifurcation. This is in contrast to carotid atherosclerosis which causes stenosis typically within 1–1.5 cm of the carotid bifurcation. Carotid atherosclerosis can also be calcified, usually absent in dissection.

3 CT angiography for intracerebral hemorrhage

CTA can identify vascular lesions as a culprit for ICH. These include:

☐ Arteriovenous malformations (AVM)

☐ Neoplasm (primary or metastatic)

☐ Venous thrombosis

☐ Reversible cerebral vasoconstriction syndrome

☐ Aneurysm

Below is an example of a ruptured AVM resulting in a left lobar hemorrhage (Fig. 6.8). Without CTA, you may suspect amyloid angiopathy as the etiology of the lobar hemorrhage. It is important as this vascular lesion may be amenable to radiosurgery.

CTA spot sign

In patients with acute intracerebral hemorrhage, hematoma expansion occurs in about 40% of patients who are scanned early, and is an independent predictor of neurological deterioration and mortality. The spot sign refers to one (or more) foci of contrast enhancement within an acute hematoma, and is predictive of ICH expansion. Patients with a CTA spot sign are at increased risk for ICH expansion and neurological deterioration due to ongoing bleeding, whereas those without a spot sign are at low risk

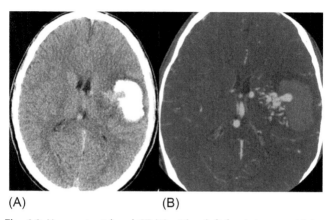

(A)   (B)

Fig. 6.8 Noncontrast head CT (A) with a left frontotemporal lobar hemorrhage. On CT angiogram (B) an AVM is identified.

for further ICH expansion. Other CT imaging markers are also being studied for their prognostic utility.

To identify the spot sign you look at the CTA source images for a focus of enhancement. Below we will review an example of the CTA spot sign in the acute stroke setting (Fig. 6.9).

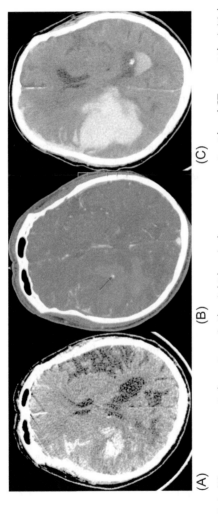

Fig. 6.9 In (A), we see an acute hematoma in the right hemisphere on noncontrast head CT scan at the initial presentation. (B) is an axial CTA (source image) showing a focus of enhancement in the acute hematoma *(red arrow)*—CTA spot sign. (C) is a noncontrast head CT 24 h after presentation revealing an increase in the size of the hematoma with mass effect, midline shift and intraventricular extension.

Summary

We reviewed an approach to CTA for acute ischemic stroke with examples of intracranial artery occlusions amenable to EVT, and examples of cerebral venous thrombosis that can be identified by CT venography. CTA also plays an important role in helping to determine stroke and TIA etiology, e.g. by identifying atherosclerotic disease, dissection, or other vasculopathies. Remember, many etiologies will be missed by carotid ultrasound. And finally, the CTA is helpful in the assessment of patients with acute ICH by identifying a potential vascular lesion or spot sign—a predictor of hematoma expansion.

In the next chapter, we will review CT perfusion, the newest frontier in code stroke imaging.

Reference

1. Tsantilas P, et al. Stroke risk in the early period after carotid related symptoms: a systematic review. *J Cardiovasc Surg*. 2015;56(6):845–852.

Further reading

2. Kamal N, Hill MD, Blacquiere DP, Boulanger JM, et al. Rapid assessment and treatment of transient ischemic attacks and minor stroke in Canadian emergency departments: Time for a paradigm shift. *Stroke*. 2015;46:2987–2990.

3. Wein T, Lindsay MP, Côté R, et al. Canadian stroke best practice recommendations: Secondary prevention of stroke, sixth edition practice guidelines, update 2017. *Int J Stroke*. 2017 Jan.

4. A practical stroke risk calculator for patients with symptomatic carotid artery stenosis is available at: https://www.ndcn.ox.ac.uk/divisions/cpsd/carotid-stenosis-tool.

5. Thompson A, Kosior J, Gladstone DJ, et al. Defining the CT angiography 'spot sign' in primary intracerebral hemorrhage. *Can J Neurol Sci*. 2009;36:456–461.

6. Brinjikji W, Krings T. *Imaging in Neurovascular Disease. A Case-Based Approach*. 1st ed. Thieme Publishers; 2020.

7. Chaturvedi S, Sacco RL. How recent data have impacted the treatment of internal carotid artery stenosis. *J Am Coll Cardiol*. 2015;65:1134–1143.

CHAPTER 7

Stroke imaging: CT perfusion

> This chapter is a brief introduction to CT perfusion (CTP). We provide a clinical framework to understand CTP such that as a practitioner you can begin to use this powerful tool to aid your acute treatment decisions. Specifically, we will discuss:
> ❏ An overview of CTP and how it supplements acute stroke imaging.
> ❏ An appreciation of assumptions made by CTP algorithms.
> ❏ A conceptual framework for understanding CTP imaging with clinical application and imaging examples.

CTP, essentially a color map of brain blood flow, is an imaging tool to estimate the presence and extent of ischemia vs infarction. The infarct **"core"** is the tissue that has already undergone infarction. Tissue that is ischemic but not yet infarcted is termed the **"penumbra."** Without reperfusion, the ischemic penumbra will eventually progress to complete infarction. In patients imaged early after stroke onset, there may be a substantial area of penumbra relative to the core, indicating brain tissue that is potentially salvageable if blood flow can be restored in time.

Fundamentally, CTP refers to how blood flows at the capillary level and this data is extracted through perfusion of dye that is performed as a contrast injection after the

The Code Stroke Handbook
https://doi.org/10.1016/B978-0-12-820522-8.00007-7

conventional CT angiogram. This allows for the estimation of cerebral blood flow, cerebral blood volume, and mean transit time, which we will discuss shortly. Often CTP is not needed following the CTA, for example, when hemorrhage is seen on noncontrast head CT, when there is clearly an already large established infarct visible on noncontrast CT, or other instances where it is otherwise unlikely to change management.

Considerable variety exists in protocols for CTP scanning and processing of the perfusion maps. Recently, standardization of tools to characterize perfusion has had a pivotal role in identifying candidates for EVT in the late time window (between 6 and 24 h poststroke onset). The algorithms utilized for this particular case (in the DEFUSE3 and DAWN clinical trials) used the RAPID software but there are other algorithms available that compute CTP maps.

MRI perfusion studies also exist, however its description is beyond the scope of this chapter.

Framework for understanding CT perfusion

CTP is described by three key parameters:
- ❏ CBF (cerebral blood flow)
- ❏ CBV (cerebral blood volume)
- ❏ MTT (mean transit time)

Cerebral blood volume is defined as the total volume of blood flowing through a volume of the brain (mL/100 g of brain tissue). **Cerebral blood flow** is defined by the volume of blood moving through a volume of brain per unit time (mL/100 g/s). **Mean transit time** is defined as the average transit time of blood, for a given brain region measured in units of time (seconds

or minutes). Core and penumbra have had different defi-
nitions over time. Previously core was defined as CBV,
but the newer measures **define core as CBF below a
certain threshold**. This is based on research that suggests that CBF is a more optimal parameter for assessing
infarct core. Similarly, MTT could be used to define a
penumbra, and a more sensitive measure of that is **Tmax**
(i.e., time to peak (TTP)), which is an index of time
from the beginning of injection of bolus contrast to
maximum enhancement (in seconds).

CTP is a dynamic measure and involves intravenous contrast administration, and this contrast is tracked with serial
imaging during its "first pass" circulation through the brain
tissue capillary bed. To calculate perfusion, there are a few assumptions that are made, one is that perfusion tracer is not dif-
fusible, metabolized or absorbed by the tissue. This is generally
felt to be the case in the normal brain, however in the context
of injury (i.e., stroke), there is a breakdown of the blood-brain
barrier and therefore this assumption does not fully hold true.
Generally, this results in an overestimation of the CT CBV.

Some practical considerations and assumptions that
CTP imaging requires are that the patient has good cardiac
output, is in normal sinus rhythm, and the absence of significant extracranial artery stenosis. During the calculation
of CTP parameters, areas of interest have to be selected and
these form the underpinnings of the arterial and venous
time density curves. Qualitative assessment of these density
curves also provides information with regards to the efficacy of the contrast injection. Furthermore, CTP imaging
relies on some thresholds that are computational in nature
and at times predetermined and thus these can result in
errors in estimating the core and penumbra.

CTP is most useful in hemispheric infarcts, such as MCA territory and in the case of scanners that are able to look at more caudal regions such as the brain stem and cerebellum. However, it is important to note that most of the validated studies of CTP are focused on the MCA territories and the posterior fossa is currently not validated. By corollary, smaller infarcts such as lacunar infarcts are not well visualized on CTP maps.

CTP can help in the assessment of stroke mimics. For example, seizures may result in maps that show the opposite of stroke, such as hyperemia with increased perfusion during an ictal state.

> Conceptually it is easy to think about cerebral blood flow as the ratio of cerebral blood volume moving across time, therefore;
>
> $$CBF = CBV/MTT$$
>
> We will use this relationship to understand the physiology of ischemic stroke and how this computes to the CTP images obtained.

In the setting of an ischemic stroke, there is intracranial vascular occlusion. This results in an increase in MTT and is affected by the degree of collateral supply to the affected area. Cerebral autoregulation results in vasodilation of the arteries distal to the occlusion and increased oxygen extraction from the blood. As a result, CBV increases, therefore CBF is either maintained or just slightly decreased (because $CBF = \uparrow CBV/\uparrow MTT$). However, as time passes there is a limit to vasodilation and further increases in MTT (compounded by tissue injury at the cellular level) result in a marked decrease in CBF.

When the CBF falls below the ischemic threshold, tissue begins to infarct.

There are important perfusion patterns to recognize in the acute stroke setting—*matched* and *mismatched* patterns. The size of the matched defect and the degree of mismatch can help guide treatment decision-making for EVT and/or tPA. In addition to the pattern of perfusion abnormality, you should describe what anatomical brain areas are at risk, as this is also an important factor for deciding about EVT or tPA.

> **A predominantly <u>matched perfusion pattern</u> occurs in areas of the brain where an <u>infarct has completed</u>, resulting in ↓CBF, and ↓CBV with ongoing ↑MTT**. In other words, this pattern reflects core and no penumbra.

This condition or rather end point is a pattern consistent with loss of sufficient perfusion to neurons and can be thought of as an irreversible loss of function corresponding with neuronal death. These patients would likely not benefit from revascularization with either tPA and/or endovascular therapy. Certainly, there are limits to CTP, and tissue identified as infarct core may have aspects that are still salvageable.

Fig. 7.1 is an example of a predominantly matched perfusion pattern. The scale is on the right—red indicates an increase and blue a decrease. In this example, in the left hemisphere, there is a decrease in CBF, a decrease in CBV, and an increase in MTT. The Tmax series is very sensitive to detect slow blood flow (i.e., prolonged MTTs) and corresponds to the time to maximum residual function.

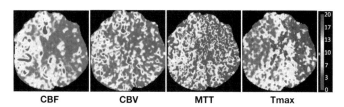

CBF   **CBV**   **MTT**   **Tmax**

Fig. 7.1 Left M1 occlusion resulting in a predominantly matched perfusion pattern.

This patient would likely not benefit from recanalization therapy as the tissue has infarcted and is at an increased risk of secondary hemorrhagic transformation.

However, if there is a mismatch pattern, then there may be salvageable brain tissue.

A predominantly <u>mismatched perfusion pattern</u> occurs in areas of the brain where there is <u>salvageable tissue</u> (ischemic but not yet infarcted), resulting in ↓ CBF, but normal CBV, and ↑ MTT.

These patients are the ideal candidates for revascularization therapy.

You will notice that the difference between a mismatched and matched perfusion pattern is CBV, which is <u>normal in a mismatch pattern</u> and <u>decreased in a matched pattern</u>.

Fig. 7.2 is an example of a predominantly mismatched perfusion pattern in a left MCA stroke. In this example, in the left hemisphere, there is a decrease in CBF, a relatively normal CBV, and an increase in MTT. The Tmax series is very sensitive to detect slow blood flow (i.e., prolonged MTTs) and corresponds to the time to maximum residual function.

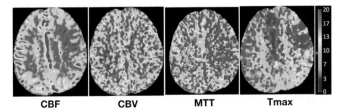

Fig. 7.2 Left MCA stroke with a predominantly mismatched perfusion pattern.

Here is a table summarizing the above acute stroke perfusion patterns. Of course, there are many different degrees of core and penumbra that can be seen. The relative change between each parameter is depicted as time progresses and tissue changes from penumbra to the core. This table is handy to keep around to easily refer back to.

Tissue region	CBF	CBV	MTT	Findings on noncontrast head CT
Penumbra ("mismatch")	Decreased	Normal (or slightly increased)	Increased	Normal, or early ischemic changes
Core ("matched")	Decreased	Decreased	Increased	Early or subacute ischemic changes

We will go through a few case examples with clinical vignettes.

Case presentation

A 79-year-old gentleman was well at 13:10 when he had a normal telephone conversation with his daughter. When she returned home at 15:15 she found him unable to speak and EMS was activated.

On arrival in the ED, he is mute with preserved comprehension. NIHSS score is 5 (mute and unable to answer the level of consciousness questions).

Suspecting an acute aphasic stroke (probably left cerebral), he is rushed to CT.

Stroke protocol imaging with head CT/CTA/CTP is completed. Noncontrast head CT and CTA are both unremarkable. CTP images are shown below (Fig. 7.3). In the left inferior frontal lobe (Broca's area), CBF is decreased (red arrow), CBV is normal, MTT is increased and the Tmax series corresponds to the time to maximum residual function indicating a mismatched perfusion pattern.

He is urgently treated with intravenous tPA at 16:20 (3 h 10 min from symptom onset).

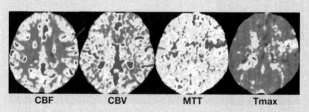

CBF   CBV   MTT   Tmax

Fig. 7.3 Left Broca's area perfusion defect.

Case presentation

A 77-year-old woman notices that she has difficulty reading the left side of the newspaper in the morning. She initially thought there was a problem with her glasses prescription and went first to her optometrist who then sent her to the emergency department. She has a past medical history of hypertension, dyslipidemia, and cataract surgery 2 months ago.

The patient describes trouble seeing out of the left side of her left eye (she is only able to appreciate the temporal field defect in the left eye) but examination reveals a left homonymous hemianopsia.

The stroke protocol imaging is obtained. The noncontrast head CT reveals hypoattenuation in the right occipital lobe. CT angiogram does not reveal an arterial occlusion. CT perfusion (CBV and MTT) is shown below (Fig. 7.4). On the CBV maps, we see decreased cerebral blood flow in the right occipital lobe and corresponding increased mean transit time MTT. CBF maps showed decreased CBF (not shown). This pattern is consistent with a mostly matched perfusion defect and corresponds to the patient's subacute presentation. She was deemed not a candidate for acute therapy.

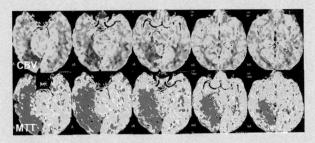

Fig. 7.4 Right occipital perfusion maps.

Some centers have transitioned to the automatic calculation of core and penumbra volumes using different software, one of which is RAPID by iSchemaView.

With more streamlined algorithms such as RAPID, which not only demonstrate an area of core/infarct as CBF < 30% (depicted in purple), and penumbra expressed as Tmax > 6 s (depicted in green), but also provide additional maps with gradations of both cerebral blood flow and Tmax, such that the provider can consider various thresholds, in the context of the individual patient, in order to assess whether the perfusion map is accurately reflecting a perfusion abnormality (Fig. 7.5).

The greatest utility of CTP is for assessment of patients presenting in the late time windows, specifically from 6 to 24 h, or when there is an unknown/unwitnessed time of stroke onset such as a wake-up stroke. For the late time window, there are specific criteria to determine whether the region of mismatch qualifies for revascularization. In general, the mismatch ratio of penumbra to the core (expressed in mL for volume) should be greater than 1.8.

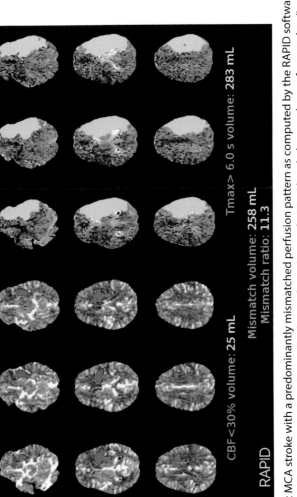

RAPID

CBF<30% volume: 25 mL

Tmax> 6.0 s volume: 283 mL

Mismatch volume: **258 mL**
Mismatch ratio: **11.3**

Fig. 7.5 Left MCA stroke with a predominantly mismatched perfusion pattern as computed by the RAPID software (by iSchemaView). Note computation of a small volume of core (in *purple*, 25 mL) and a large volume of penumbra (in *green*, 283 mL) with a mismatch volume. For specific criteria for mismatch in the 6–24 time window, refer to local protocols or guidelines as there may be variations in the recommended inclusion and exclusion criteria.

CTP considerations and pitfalls

With the advent of algorithmic computation of CTP maps and their readily available nature during a code stroke, there can be a tendency to use these maps to make a clinical decision without thinking more deeply about what the perfusion maps actually show. During a code stroke, one must stay vigilant and attentive to the details of what CT perfusion is showing in the context of the patient but also about what the analysis actually shows.

CTP makes a series of assumptions, both at the technical level and also about the patient's hemodynamics. Furthermore, there are other technical factors such as the movement of the patient and the quality and timing of the contrast injection. If all of these are minimized and optimized, to understand a CTP map one still needs to deploy some understanding of what is actually being shown on the perfusion maps. Lastly, the use of CTP has primarily been validated in patient selection for EVT. Caution should be used when interpreting CTP for decisions about tPA, as clinical trials of thrombolysis did not utilize this modality.

Summary

In this chapter, we have discussed a framework to understand CTP and how the physiology is reflected in the metrics computed in perfusion imaging. CTP imaging is the most recent biomarker in acute stroke imaging that allows estimation of a core and penumbra and their relative mismatch, which is especially helpful in the extended 6–24 h time windows. Furthermore, we outlined some of the assumptions and important considerations that are relevant to CTP, which inform the reader of its limitations and utility.

Further reading

1. Allmendinger AM, Tang ER, Lui YW, Spektor V. Imaging of stroke: part 1, perfusion CT—overview of imaging technique, interpretation peraks, and common pitfalls. *AJR Am J Roentgenol.* 2012;198(1):52–62.
2. Brinjikji W, Krings T. *Imaging in Neurovascular Disease. A Case-Based Approach.* 1st ed. Thieme Publishers; 2020.
3. Lui YW, Tang ER, Allmendinger AM, Spektor V. Evaluation of CT perfusion in the setting of cerebral ischemia: patterns and pitfalls. *Am J Neuroradiol.* 2010;31(9):1552–1563.

CHAPTER 8

Acute ischemic stroke treatment: Alteplase

In the next series of chapters we will provide you with an organized approach to emergency reperfusion treatments for acute ischemic stroke: intravenous thrombolysis with alteplase (tPA) and endovascular therapy (EVT). We will discuss acute blood pressure management and the indications for acute treatment with single or dual antiplatelet therapy for patients not receiving tPA or EVT.

In this chapter, we will discuss IV tPA—patient selection, administration pearls, and pitfalls.

Before we discuss thrombolytic therapy, it is humbling and insightful to see how far acute stroke care has advanced over the past 50 years.

Progress in acute stroke care over the past 50 years

1969—First CT scanner
1977—First MRI scanner
1995—NINDS trial—established 3-h window for tPA
2008—ECASS III trial—established 4.5-h window for tPA

(Continued)

2015—EVT becomes standard of care with 5 positive trials (MR CLEAN, ESCAPE, SWIFT PRIME, REVASCAT, EXTEND IA)
2017—DAWN and DIFFUSE 3 trials—extended window for EVT up to 24 h
2018/2019—WAKE-UP STROKE and EXTEND trials—extended tPA window up to 9 h for highly selected patients

1 Intravenous thrombolysis: efficacy and patient selection

Alteplase, a tissue plasminogen activator (tPA), catalyzes the conversion of plasminogen to plasmin, the enzyme responsible for the breakdown of fibrin. The Food and Drug Administration (FDA) approved alteplase for the treatment of acute ischemic stroke in 1996, after the publication of the landmark NINDS trial (see below). In Canada, tPA was licensed by Health Canada in 1999 (conditional approval) and 2002 (full approval) for eligible patients who can be treated with the first 3 h of stroke onset.

Currently, intravenous tPA is guideline-recommended for eligible patients with disabling ischemic stroke who can be treated within 4.5 h of stroke onset.

Two landmark tPA stroke trials

The **NINDS trial**[1] was a randomized, double-blind trial of intravenous tPA compared with placebo. It showed benefit in patients treated within a 3-h window from the onset. Patients treated with tPA within 3 h of stroke onset were at least 30% more likely to have a favorable outcome at 3 months. Symptomatic intracerebral hemorrhage (within 36 h after stroke onset) occurred in approximately 6% of patients treated with tPA as compared with 0.6% among those given placebo. There was no difference in mortality between the two groups.

A positive pooled analysis led to the **ECASS III trial**[2] showing tPA administered between <u>3 and 4.5 h</u> after onset increases the rate of favorable outcome compared with placebo. Like NINDS, there was a higher incidence of intracerebral hemorrhage and no difference in mortality between the two groups.

More recently, two new trials have shown benefit of tPA within an extended time window (up to 9 h post-onset) in highly selected patients based on strict imaging criteria (CT perfusion or MRI). We will discuss these two trials at the end of the tPA section.

The **number needed to treat (NNT)** is a measure used to quantify the success of an intervention and to compare different interventions.

Below is the NNT for tPA for acute ischemic stroke derived from a meta-analysis of nine randomized phase-3 trials involving 6757 patients.[3,13]

Benefits of tPA for acute ischemic stroke

The NNT for one additional patient to have an excellent functional outcome from tPA at 90 days (defined as mRS 0–1★) is **time dependent.** Below is the NNT based on the time from stroke onset to initiation of tPA:

- ❏ < 3 h: NNT = 10
- ❏ 3–4.5 h: NNT = 19

(Continued)

*mRS = modified Rankin scale. mRS 0 = fully recovered; mRS 1 = symptoms but no disability; mRS 0–2 = independent functional outcome; mRS 3–5 = disability and dependency; mRS 6 = death.

Another way to express the benefit of tPA is by considering improvement as any reduction in disability level across the entire range of the mRS. According to an analysis of the NINDS trial by Saver,[4] tPA reduced disability in approximately one in three patients treated. In other words, for every 100 patients treated with tPA, on average 32 patients had a better final outcome as a result of treatment (improvement by one or more disability grades on the 7-point mRS) and three had a worse final outcome.

1.1 Time to treatment

It is important to remember that tPA is a highly time-sensitive treatment. The benefit of tPA treatment decreases markedly as time elapses from the onset of the stroke to tPA administration. Early treatment is more likely to reduce the degree of neurological impairment and disability. The recommended target treatment time is < 30 min from hospital arrival. Every minute counts in the assessment and treatment of patients with acute stroke—think speed! As stated by Dr. Hill and Coutts[5]: "*Doctors treating patients who have had an acute ischemic stroke must feel the need for speed more feverishly than a racing driver.*"

Recanalization and reperfusion are the goals of acute stroke treatment and an important concept to understand is collateral blood flow. Neurons can potentially be rescued with timely intervention but individual patient outcomes depend on the degree of collateral blood flow to the affected area between time of stroke onset and treatment. Collateral blood flow can come from branches of the external carotid artery, the circle of Willis, or small leptomeningeal arteries. It is tenuous and can only help for a limited amount of time before the penumbra (area of ischemic but potentially salvageable brain tissue) progresses to irreversible infarction. There is considerable variation in collateral blood flow between individual patients, which provides the rationale for individualized treatments and longer treatment time windows in selected patients.

1.2 Stroke severity

tPA should be considered for patients who have neurological deficits that are predicted to be disabling to the patient if they persist. However, as mentioned in Chapter 3, the numerical NIHSS score does not always correlate with degree of disability so treatment decisions need to be individualized. The type of deficit and individual characteristics of the patient (impact on work, hobbies, driving, hand dominance, etc.) must be taken into consideration. For example, isolated homonymous hemianopia can render an individual ineligible to drive, neglect and aphasia can have low NIHSS score but be very disabling, leg weakness may preclude walking, and hand weakness (especially the dominant hand) may have a significant impact on a person's daily functioning.

1.3 How to administer tPA at the bedside

The standard North American dose of alteplase for stroke is 0.9 mg/kg (max 90 mg total dose). A 10% intravenous bolus is pushed over 1 min and the remainder is infused over 1 h. In some hospitals, the infusion pump will also administer the bolus. Note that the dose of alteplase for acute stroke is lower than the dose used for acute myocardial infarction. For dose calculations, measure the patient's body weight (if not possible, use patient/family self-report or best estimate).

After tPA is given the patient should be closely monitored. It is essential to maintain blood pressure under 180/105 for 24 hours post–tPA to minimize the risk of tPA-related intracerebral hemorrhage. See blood pressure chapter for further details (Chapter 11). If there is clinical concern for bleeding then the tPA infusion should be immediately stopped, and an urgent noncontrast CT head should be obtained if intracranial hemorrhage is suspected. To minimize the risk of bleeding, it is recommended to avoid antiplatelet and anticoagulant therapy within the first 24 hours post-tPA.

It is always good practice to discuss the stroke diagnosis and the treatment options (rationale, benefits, risks, alternatives) to the patient or family as part of the informed consent process. As tPA is the standard care treatment for eligible patients with acute ischemic stroke, procedures for emergency consent apply if the patient is unable to provide consent and if a legally authorized representative is not available.

If tPA is not being administered, it is important to document why. We recommend explaining to patients and families that the patient was assessed for tPA (same applies for EVT) and clearly outline (and document) the reason(s) why the patient was not a candidate for tPA or why tPA was not recommended.

If tPA is not being administered because stroke symptoms appear too mild or the patient appears to be rapidly improving, we recommend keeping the patient under close observation and conducting repeated neurological assessments within the 4.5 hour time window to reassess in case the stroke deficits worsen. It is not uncommon for stroke symptoms to fluctuate in severity during the evolution of an acute stroke. Studies show that among patients for whom tPA is withheld because of rapidly improving symptomatology, about one-third will subsequently worsen. Therefore, be careful not to be falsely reassured by symptoms that appear to be improving spontaneously, and do not rely on a single time–point assessment to exclude patients from tPA.

Case presentation

A 62-year-old woman was having dinner with her children when she suddenly could not speak and could not lift her right arm. Her family also noticed a facial droop. Her son immediately called 911 and she was transported to the emergency department. Her symptoms started 45 min ago. She has hypertension and smokes a pack a day of cigarettes.

On initial assessment, her blood pressure is 176/89 mmHg and she is in atrial fibrillation. Her NIHSS score is 9 (2 points for right facial weakness, 2 points for right arm weakness, 1 point for right leg weakness, 1 point for sensory impairment, 1 point for dysarthria, and 2 points for aphasia).

Noncontrast CT head is negative for hemorrhage, hyperdense vessel sign or loss of gray-white differentiation (ASPECTS = 10). CT angiogram reveals a distal left M2 branch occlusion. No extracranial or intracranial carotid artery stenosis. The CT brain perfusion study shows a good mismatch pattern within the left MCA territory.

The diagnosis is an embolic acute ischemic stroke. The most likely etiology is cardioembolism from atrial fibrillation. Her neurological deficits are disabling. She is a good candidate for tPA. She meets all clinical and imaging criteria and has no known contraindications. She is within the time window and has a favorable imaging profile. All emergency stroke treatment options were considered: IV tPA, EVT, antiplatelet therapy. She is not a candidate for EVT as her M2 clot is too distal to be reached by a catheter.

tPA is indicated and recommended to give her the best chance for improvement and avoidance of disability. The diagnosis and treatment options were explained to her and her family, including the potential for tPA-related bleeding complications that could be serious or fatal (including ICH). In her case, the benefits of tPA were felt to outweigh the risks of bleeding complications. Her family understood the issues and agreed with the proposed treatment.

She was treated with tPA as per standard protocol. The bolus was administered at 1 h 15 min from symptom onset, followed by a 1 h infusion. She was admitted to a closely monitored unit for standard post-tPA management.

The next day on assessment her NIHSS score improved to 3. After her 24-h head CT scan was done and showed no hemorrhage daily low-dose aspirin was started. After 7 days, her aspirin was stopped and she was started on a direct oral anticoagulant for secondary stroke prevention given her diagnosis of atrial fibrillation. On day 8 she was discharged home with a plan for outpatient rehabilitation and outpatient clinic follow-up.

1.4 tPA complications

The main risk of tPA is bleeding, either systemic or intracranial. The risk of tPA-related symptomatic intracranial hemorrhage (sICH) is approximately **2%–6%** (vs 0.4% with placebo), which can be quoted to patients and their families when discussing the benefits and risks of tPA. Of the tPA-related intracranial hemorrhages that do occur, many are bleeds into large infarcts that would otherwise have caused substantial disability.

Risk factors for tPA-related symptomatic ICH include:
❏ Large stroke (high NIHSS score) or extensive acute ischemic changes on CT (i.e., low ASPECTS score)

❏ Older age
❏ Hyperglycemia
❏ Uncontrolled hypertension

There is no standard treatment protocol for reversal of tPA, and protocols differ between hospitals. One protocol consists of giving cryoprecipitate (or fibrinogen) plus tranexamic acid. As well, urgent blood should be drawn for CBC, platelet count, PTT, fibrinogen, INR and type, and cross. Intensive care, hematology, and neurosurgery should be consulted urgently as needed.

Harms of tPA for acute ischemic stroke[13]

The number of patients needed to treat with tPA for one patient to be harmed (NNH) in terms of a fatal intracerebral hemorrhage is:

❏ < 3 h: NNH = 40
❏ 3–4.5 h: NNH = 50
❏ 4.5–6 h: NNH = 40

Less common but important complications from tPA include angioedema (1.3%), and anaphylaxis (0.5%). The risk of angioedema is higher in patients taking angiotensin-converting enzyme (ACE) inhibitors, and can compromise the airway.

You can treat hypersensitivity/angioedema with antihistamines, steroids, and standard airway management. The protocol may differ between hospitals, but a typical hospital protocol consists of methylprednisolone 125 mg IV, diphenhydramine 50 mg IV, and ranitidine 50 mg IV.

1.5 tPA contraindications

There are absolute and relative contraindications to tPA that are important to screen for prior to treatment. Below is a table from the Canadian guidelines. You may wish to keep this table handy during a code stroke for quick reference.

Contraindications to tPA

Absolute exclusion criteria:
- ❏ Any source of active bleeding or bleeding diathesis
- ❏ Any hemorrhage on brain imaging

Relative exclusion criteria:*
Historical
- ❏ History of intracranial hemorrhage
- ❏ Stroke or serious head or spinal trauma in the preceding 3 months
- ❏ Magor surgery, such as cardiac, thoracic, abdominal or orthopedic in the preceding 2 weeks
- ❏ Arterial puncture at a noncompressible site in the previous 7 days

Clinical
- ❏ Symptoms suggestive of subarachnoid hemorrhage
- ❏ Stroke symptoms due to another nonischemic acute neurological condition such as seizure with postictal Todd's paralysis or focal neurological signs due to severe hypo- or hyperglycemia
- ❏ Hypertension refractory to aggressive hyperacute antihypertensive treatment such that target blood pressure less than 185/110 mmHg cannot be achieved or maintained

(Continued)

❏ Patient currently prescribed and taking a direct non-vitamin K oral anticoagulant (Apixaban, Rivaroxaban, Dabigatran)

Neuroimaging
❏ CT showing early signs of extensive infarction

Laboratory
❏ INR > 1.7
❏ Platelets < 100
❏ Glucose < 2.7 mmol/L, or > 22 mmol/L
❏ Elevated activated partial-thromboplastin time (aPTT)

★The relative contraindications require clinical judgment based on the specific situation (we will discuss a few individually below).

Boulanger JM, et al. Canadian stroke best practice recommendations for acute stroke management: prehospital, emergency department, and acute inpatient stroke care, 6th edition, update 2018. *Int J Stroke*. 2018;139:949–984.

Below we will review the relative contraindications to tPA and what factors to consider when weighing the benefits and risks on a case-by-case basis.

History of intracerebral hemorrhage

There are sparse data on giving tPA to patients with a prior history of ICH. Of the handful of published cases in which tPA was given "off-label" for patients with prior ICH, the outcomes were favorable. Individual factors may influence the benefit/risk balance such as the time elapsed since the prior ICH, etiology of previous ICH, and whether there was definitive treatment (i.e., coiling or clipping for aneurysmal subarachnoid hemorrhage), if they have a history of cerebral microbleeds (especially more than 10), and volume and location of residual encephalomalacia.

Ischemic stroke within the previous 3 months

The safety of tPA for such patients is largely unknown and there are limited published data available. You may consider it by weighing individual patient characteristics such as severity of current stroke, size, and mechanism of previous infarction, and age of the patient.

Recent major surgery in preceding 2 weeks or arterial puncture of noncompressible vessel in preceding 7 days

The category of "major surgery" includes cardiac, thoracic, abdominal, or orthopedic surgery in the preceding 2 weeks. There are sparse data for these patients and there may be a component of a reporting bias. The risk of giving tPA to these patients is hemorrhage in the recent surgical area. There are few cases in the literature of systemic hemorrhages or bleeding at the site of recent surgery after tPA was given, that required invasive interventions.

Arterial puncture of a noncompressible vessel within 7 days includes patients with the placement of cardiac pacing or defibrillation leads, dialysis catheters, or placement of transcatheter heart valves. These patients may be in the intensive care unit and have other factors related to their illness that increase their risk of bleeding.

Seizure at onset

Seizures can occur at the onset of an ischemic stroke. The rationale for including it as a relative contraindication is to avoid giving tPA to a stroke mimic, i.e., a seizure with a postictal deficit, in the absence of an acute stroke.

There are more than 300 published cases of tPA given to patients presenting with ischemic stroke and seizure at onset, with only a handful of patients with symptomatic ICH. CTA can be helpful here. When clinical and radiographic presentation support seizure secondary to acute ischemic stroke (especially if CTA shows a vessel occlusion), then tPA (and/or EVT) should be considered.

Patient on a direct (non-vitamin K) oral anticoagulant (apixaban, dabigatran, edoxaban, rivaroxaban)

The safety of thrombolysis in patients taking direct oral anticoagulants (DOACs) is uncertain and it may be harmful. As a general rule, if the patient took their last dose of a DOAC within the last 48 h, then it is typically considered a contraindication to tPA. A careful history often elicited from family members or investigating the patient's blister pack may help gather this information.

Case presentation

An 88-year-old man was on the phone with his daughter when he started to slur his words and could not hold the phone in his left hand. His wife noticed a facial droop. She immediately called 911. He has atrial fibrillation and his anticoagulation was recently held because of a left subdural hematoma that occurred 1 month ago after a fall on the stairs.

On initial assessment, his blood pressure is 205/100 mmHg and he is in atrial fibrillation. His NIHSS score is 6 (2 points for left facial weakness, 1 point for left arm weakness, 1 point for sensory loss, 1 point for dysarthria and 1 point for neglect).

Noncontrast CT head reveals a subacute moderate size left subdural hematoma, no hyperdense vessel sign, and loss of gray-white differentiation in the right M6 region (ASPECTS = 9). CT angiogram shows a right M2 clot too distal for EVT.

Given the presence of intracranial blood, tPA is too risky and is contraindicated. This was explained to him and his family. He was admitted to the stroke unit for standard stroke management and rehabilitation.

1.6 Special considerations

tPA for lacunes

As mentioned in Chapter 4 (Stroke Syndromes), lacunar infarcts can occur anywhere from the centrum semiovale to the basis pontis, and clinically present with classic lacunar syndromes. There has been some debate regarding the efficacy of tPA for lacunar infarcts, given the underlying mechanism is small vessel disease (in the majority) rather than an embolic phenomenon.

The literature provides evidence that patients with lacunar infarcts still benefit from tPA in terms of better functional outcomes, on average, as compared with those who do not receive tPA. Patients with severe chronic small vessel disease may have a higher risk of symptomatic ICH with tPA, although this does not off-set the benefit they may receive from tPA.

tPA for minor strokes

The decision to administer tPA to patients presenting with very mild and non-disabling deficits is challenging and currently controversial. The **PRISMS trial**[6] compared tPA vs aspirin in patients with NIHSS of 0–5, whose deficits would not prevent them from performing basic activities. The study found no significant difference in favorable outcomes with tPA in this population, but the trial was terminated early, limiting any definitive conclusions, and did not require patients to have a vessel occlusion on CTA. The presence of a vessel occlusion on CTA or large vascular territory at risk on CTP imaging, may be helpful for this decision-making for tPA. The TEMPO-2 trial is investigating this question further.

Extended tPA time window

In 2018 and 2019 two trials provided evidence that tPA treatment can be extended up to 9h in highly selected patients using very specific imaging criteria. The Wake-Up Stroke trial[7] showed that a mismatch between diffusion-weighted imaging and FLAIR sequence on MRI (DWI positive, FLAIR negative), could be used to administer tPA to patients with an unknown time of symptom onset. The rationale was that this imaging pattern suggested the stroke occurred within approximately 4.5h.

The Extend trial,[8] was a multicenter, randomized, placebo-controlled trial enrolling patients between 4.5 and 9h from stroke onset, or on awakening with stroke symptoms (if within 9h from the midpoint of sleep). These patients had hypoperfused but salvageable regions identified by perfusion imaging mismatch. The mismatch was defined as a ratio > 1.2 between the volume of hypoperfusion and the volume of the ischemic core, an absolute difference in volume > 10 mL, and an ischemic-core volume of < 70 mL.

tPA resulted in a higher percentage of patients with a mRS of 0 or 1 (indicating no disability) compared to placebo. There were more cases of symptomatic ICH in the tPA group (~6% vs 1%). The authors concluded that in patients with favorable CT perfusion imaging, giving tPA between 4.5 and 9h resulted in a higher percentage of patients with excellent outcomes, albeit with an increased risk of ICH.

Summary of tPA

tPA is indicated for acute ischemic stroke patients with:

1. A measurable or disabling neurological deficit
2. Time window from stroke onset (or last seen normal time) is < 4.5 h, however, (emerging evidence supports administration up to 9 h if strict imaging criteria show a favorable mismatch pattern)
3. Absence of extensive acute ischemic changes on CT
4. No intracranial hemorrhage
5. No major contraindications, and blood pressure < 185/110 mmHg

The NNT for one additional patient to achieve an excellent outcome (no disability; mRS score 0–1) for tPA given < 3 h from the onset is 10, and NNT is 19 when given between 3 and 4.5 h.

There is an approximate 6% risk of symptomatic intracranial hemorrhage (2% risk of a fatal ICH) after tPA.

The only absolute contraindication to tPA is active intracranial or systemic bleeding, the remainder is relative contraindications and carefully considered on a case-by-case basis.

Summary

In this chapter, we reviewed the indication and eligibility for tPA, dosing absolute and relative contraindications, and the need for speed. The NNT and NNH for tPA are good statistics to remember to quote to patients and families when discussing the rationale, benefits, risks and alternatives for tPA. We also reviewed special considerations, such as giving tPA for lacunes, minor strokes, and the extended time-window up to 9 h based on imaging criteria.

References and Further Reading

1. National Institute of Neurological Disorders and Stroke rt-PA Stroke Study Group. Tissue plasminogen activator for acute ischemic stroke. *N Engl J Med.* 1995;333(24):1581–1587.
2. Hacke W, et al. Thrombolysis with alteplase 3 to 4.5 hours after acute ischemic stroke. *N Engl J Med.* 2008;359(13):1317–1329.
3. Emberson J, et al. Effect of treatment delay, age and stroke severity on the effects of intravenous thrombolysis with alteplase for acute ischaemic stroke: a meta-analysis of individual patient data from randomised trials. *Lancet.* 2014;384(99958):1929–1935.
4. Saver JL. Number needed to treat estimates incorporating effects over the entire range of clinical outcomes: novel derivation method and application to thrombolytic therapy for acute stroke. *Arch Neurol.* 2004;61(7):1066–1070.
5. Hill MD, Coutts SB. Alteplase in acute ischaemic stroke: the need for speed. *Lancet.* 2014;384(9958):1904–1906.
6. Khatri P, Kleindorfer DO, Devlin T, et al. Effect of Alteplase vs Aspirin on functional outcome for patients with acute ischemic stroke and minor nondisabling neurologic deficits.The PRISMS Randomized Clinical Trial. *JAMA.* 2018;320(2):156–166.
7. Thomalla G, et al. MRI-guided thrombolysis for stroke with unknown time of onset. *N Engl J Med.* 2018;379(7):611–622.
8. Ma H, et al. Thrombolysis guided by perfusion imaging up to 9 hours after onset of stroke. *N Engl J Med.* 2019;380(19):1795–1803.
9. Boulanger JM, et al. Canadian stroke best practice recommendations for acute stroke management: prehospital, emergency department, and acute inpatient stroke care, 6th edition, update 2018. *Int J Stroke.* 2018;13(9):949–984.
10. Caplan LR, Biller J, Leary M, et al. *Primer on Cerebrovascular Diseases.* Academic Press; 2017.
11. Demaerschalk BM, Kleindorfer DO, Adeoye OM, et al. Scientific rationale for the inclusion and exclusion criteria for intravenous alteplase in acute ischemic stroke: a statement for healthcare professionals from the American Heart Association/American Stroke Association. *Stroke.* 2016;47(2):581–641.
12. Fugate JE, Rabinstein AA. Absolute and relative contraindications to IV rt-PA for acute ischemic stroke. *Neurohospitalist.* 2015;5(3):110–121.
13. https://www.thennt.com/nnt/thrombolytics-acute-ischemic-stroke/.
14. Pantoni L, Fierini F, Poggesi A.Thrombolysis in acute stroke patients with cerebral small vessel disease. *Cerebrovasc Dis.* 2014;37(1):5–13.
15. Rabinstein A. Treatment of acute ischemic stroke. *Continuum.* 2017;23(1):62–81.

CHAPTER 9

Acute ischemic stroke treatment: Endovascular therapy

This chapter will provide you with an overview of endovascular therapy (EVT) for large vessel occlusion strokes. We will specifically review:
- ❏ Patient selection criteria for EVT within 6 h of stroke onset.
- ❏ Patient selection criteria for EVT between 6 and 24 h of stroke onset.
- ❏ The benefit of EVT for large vessel occlusion in the anterior circulation, with a clinical case example.

EVT refers to mechanical thrombectomy (aspiration or removal with a stent-retriever catheter) or direct intraarterial or intraclot lysis. In 2015, five randomized trials convincingly demonstrated a major benefit of EVT for patients with acute stroke due to proximal anterior circulation occlusions. As such, it has become the standard of care emergency treatment for eligible patients in regions where it is available. The positive trial results were attributed to the newer generation stent-retriever technology and better patient selection based on imaging.

The Code Stroke Handbook
https://doi.org/10.1016/B978-0-12-820522-8.00009-0
© 2020 Elsevier Inc. All rights reserved.

The five trials are: MR CLEAN, ESCAPE, SWIFT PRIME, REVASCAT, and EXTEND IA. Four of the five trials were terminated early because of overwhelming treatment efficacy.

Keep in mind that EVT should generally be used in combination with intravenous tPA if the patient is a tPA candidate (although ongoing studies are investigating whether or not tPA administration is truly necessary if a patient is going directly to EVT). Of note, large proximal clots that are potentially amenable to EVT are typically more resistant to thrombolysis. On the other hand, tPA may lyse small/distal clots which are not accessible by EVT. Approximately 10% of ischemic strokes are due to a large vessel occlusion in the anterior circulation and present to hospital within 6 h.

Efficacy of endovascular therapy

Metaanalyses have confirmed the substantial benefit of EVT for improving outcomes in patients with acute stroke due to proximal large anterior circulation artery occlusions. According to pooled analysis of the 5 EVT trials involving 1287 patients,[1] endovascular thrombectomy added to best medical therapy significantly reduces disability as compared with best medical therapy alone: **endovascular therapy more than doubles the odds of achieving a favorable recovery, defined as mRS score 0–1 (no disability) or mRS score 0–2 (independent functioning), and more than triples the odds of achieving a virtually complete neurological recovery (NIHSS score 0–2 points).** In the Canadian-led ESCAPE trial, EVT increased the proportion of stroke patients surviving with a favorable outcome (Rankin score 0–2, i.e., functional independence) from 29% in the medical therapy group to 53% in the EVT group.

Below is the NNT in anterior circulation EVT for large vessel occlusion, in standard and extended time window trials.

Benefits in NNT for EVT in acute anterior circulation large vessel occlusion[4,5]

NNT from the metaanalysis of five trials (MR CLEAN, ESCAPE, SWIFT PRIME, REVASCAT, and EXTEND IA):

NNT = 2.6 for improved functional outcomes at 90 days (defined as improvement by at least one level on the mRS)

NNT = 5 for functional independence at 90 days (mRS 0–2*)

These findings were consistent across different subgroups including: age, sex, NIHSS, ASPECTS, site of intracranial occlusion, and if tPA was given.

There was no significant difference in symptomatic ICH and mortality between patients receiving EVT (± tPA) compared to only tPA.

NNT from extended time window trials (DAWN and DIFFUSE 3):

NNT = 3–4 for functional independence at 90 days

NNH = 35 (1 in 35 patients will experience a symptomatic intracranial hemorrhage)

*mRS 0–1 = excellent functional outcome; mRS 0–2 = independent functional outcome; mRS 3–4 = dependency; mRS 5 = bedbound; mRS 6 = death.

Below we highlight the patient selection criteria for EVT as per the current Canadian Stroke Best Practice Recommendations:

EVT clinical/imaging selection criteria for patients arriving <u>within 6 h</u> of stroke onset:

1. Persistent disabling stroke deficit and an NIHSS of 6 or greater,
2. Acute intracranial artery occlusion in the anterior circulation amenable to clot retrieval (which includes the distal ICA, M1, or proximal M2 division of MCA).
3. Small-to-moderate ischemic core (i.e., infarcted brain tissue), which can be estimated as an ASPECTS score of 6 or higher.

EVT clinical/imaging selection criteria for patients arriving <u>later than 6 h</u> (and < 24 h) of stroke onset:

DAWN and DEFUSE 3 trials provided evidence that highly selected patients with disabling stroke symptoms may benefit from EVT up to 24 h. This includes patients that awoke with stroke symptoms (i.e., wake-up strokes). Below are the DEFUSE 3 trial criteria.

<u>DEFUSE 3 trial criteria:</u>

1. Last seen normal between <u>6 and 16 h</u>
2. Intracranial arterial occlusion of the ICA or the M1 segment of the MCA
3. An NIHSS score of 6 or greater
4. Ischemic core volume < 70 mL, mismatch ratio 1.8 or greater, and mismatch volume 15 mL or greater
5. Age 18–90 years old

Mismatch ratio = the volume of the perfusion lesion divided by the volume of the ischemic core.
Mismatch volume = volume of perfusion lesion minus the volume of ischemic core.

Boulanger JM, et al. Canadian stroke best practice recommendations for acute stroke management: prehospital, emergency department, and acute inpatient stroke care, 6th edition, update 2018. *Int J Stroke*. 2018;13(9):949–984.

Case presentation

A 72-year-old woman was last seen well at 13:00 by her husband prior to her afternoon nap. She awoke at 14:15 with right arm weakness and decided to try and sleep it off. She awoke again at 15:30 with profound right arm and leg weakness, and when she tried to speak to her husband, she was unable to do so. He immediately called 911.

She arrives at the emergency department at 16:00 and is assessed right away. On initial assessment her blood pressure is 210/105 mmHg, heart rate of 88 bpm and regular. She is awake and alert but mute, unable to name or repeat any words, and unable to obey any simple commands. Her initial NIHSS score is 24 (1 point for LOC, 2 points for LOC questions, 2 points for LOC commands, 2 point for gaze deviation to the left, 2 points for homonymous hemianopia, 2 points for facial weakness, 4 points for right arm weakness, 4 points for right leg weakness, 2 points for sensory loss, and 3 points for aphasia).

She is rushed to CT. Noncontrast CT head reveals a hyperdense left MCA sign and loss of gray-white differentiation in the left insula, M2, and M3 (ASPECTS = 7). CT angiogram shows a proximal left M1 occlusion but reasonable collaterals. CT perfusion shows a mismatch perfusion pattern with a small ischemic core volume.

The diagnosis is a large severe acute ischemic stroke due to an embolic M1 occlusion of undetermined etiology. Without recanalization the prognosis is predicted to be very poor (global aphasia, severe disability, and dependence). The recommended treatment in this situation is tPA plus EVT to give her the best chance for improvement and avoidance of long-term disability.

After assessment and neuroimaging, it is 16:20 (3 h and 20 min from her last seen normal time). She is given labetalol 10 mg IV to lower her blood pressure to < 185/110 mmHg, followed immediately by IV tPA administration at 16:40 (door-to-needle time of 40 min). She is immediately taken to the angio suite for EVT. Groin puncture occurs at 17:15 (door-to-groin puncture time of 1 h 15 min). The EVT

(Continued)

procedure was successful in achieving complete vessel recanalization at 17:45, accompanied by dramatic neurological recovery. See picture below.

She was admitted to the intensive care unit for standard post-tPA/EVT management and blood pressure control (< 180/105 mmHg). At 24 h her NIHSS score had improved to 3 (1 point for facial droop, 1 point for right arm weakness, and 1 point for sensation). Her CT scan shows development of only a small subcortical infarct and no hemorrhage. She completes the standard etiological stroke workup and is able to be discharged 3 days later with a follow-up plan in place and referral for outpatient rehabilitation. She is prescribed aspirin 81 mg daily for secondary stroke prevention and discharged with a wearable ECG monitor to screen for paroxysmal atrial fibrillation which, if detected, may warrant anticoagulant therapy.

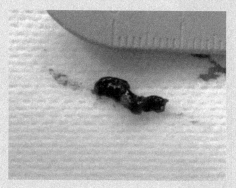

Embolic M1 clot removed by EVT (Photo courtesy of Dr. Leodante da Costa).

Imaging and treatment algorithm

To summarize the flow of the code stroke, as many tasks are completed in parallel and sequential order, we have created an imaging and treatment algorithm (Fig. 9.1). The noncontrast head CT (NCCT) and CTA are obtained consecutively, but CTP may be situation and location dependent. Blue items support a decision for thrombolysis, and purple factors support a decision of EVT. Red factors would support no hyperacute treatment.

Summary

In this chapter, we reviewed the EVT guidelines for patient selection in anterior circulation proximal large vessel occlusions in various time windows (within 6 h and extended time window up to 24 h) and the associated benefits in terms of NNT.

A good statistic to remember is, EVT for anterior circulation large vessel occlusion, within 6 h from stroke onset, has an NNT of 5 for recovery of functional independence at 90 days.

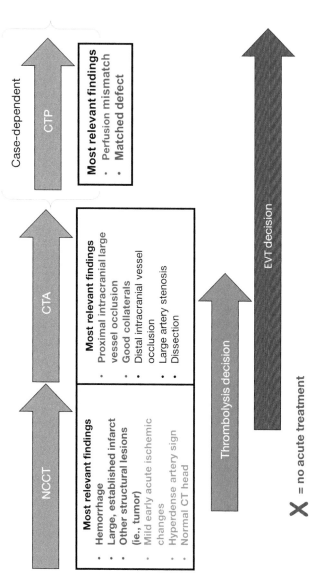

Fig. 9.1 Imaging and treatment algorithm.

References and Further Reading

1. Goyal M, et al. Endovascular thrombectomy after large-vessel ischaemic stroke: a meta-analysis of individual patient data from five randomized trials. *Lancet*. 2016;387(10029):1723–1731.
2. Albers GW, et al. Thrombectomy for stroke at 6 to 16 hours with selection by perfusion imaging. *N Engl J Med*. 2018;378(8):708–718.
3. Boulanger JM, et al. Canadian stroke best practice recommendations for acute stroke management: prehospital, emergency department, and acute inpatient stroke care, 6th edition, update 2018. *Int J Stroke*. 2018;13(9):949–984.
4. http://www.thennt.com/nnt/endovascular-thrombectomy-ischemic-stroke-beyond-6-hours-onset-symptoms/.
5. http://www.thennt.com/nnt/early-endovascular-thrombectomy-large-vessel-ischemic-stroke-reduces-disability-90-days/.
6. Noqueira RG, et al. Thrombectomy 6 to 24 hours after stroke with a mismatch between deficit and infarct. *N Engl J Med*. 2018;378(1):11–21.
7. Rabinstein A. Treatment of acute ischemic stroke. *Continuum*. 2017;23(1):62–81.

CHAPTER 10

Basilar artery occlusion

This chapter will provide you with a clinical approach to early recognition and management of basilar artery occlusions. We will review:
- ❏ Clinical syndromes associated with occlusion of the basilar artery (proximal basilar occlusion and top of the basilar).
- ❏ Management of basilar artery occlusion—current evidence for tPA and EVT.

Basilar artery occlusion (BAO) is relatively uncommon (it accounts for about 1% of ischemic strokes) but is a diagnosis you do not want to miss, given that it has the highest mortality and morbidity of any ischemic stroke type. Importantly, the time window for intervention with intravenous thrombolysis and endovascular therapy is considerably longer than it is for anterior circulation strokes. When basilar stroke is suspected, the recommended diagnostic test is an emergency head CT and CT angiogram. *Time is brain(stem)*…Without recanalization, the prognosis is usually dismal. With timely recanalization, good outcomes are possible.

Patients with acute BAO may present with sudden loss of consciousness, hemiparesis or quadriparesis or

The Code Stroke Handbook
https://doi.org/10.1016/B978-0-12-820522-8.00010-7

bulbar symptoms (dysarthria, anarthria, diplopia, vertigo, facial palsy, etc.). Another clinical presentation can be a *stuttering course of brainstem symptoms* (diplopia, dysarthria, vertigo, balance difficulty) progressing to a decreased level of consciousness. The progressive/stuttering course is often a result of severe basilar artery atherosclerotic disease. Prodromal (brainstem) symptoms may occur in up to 60% of patients who eventually present with BAO. Let us revisit the basilar artery syndromes.

Proximal basilar artery syndrome

The neurological symptoms associated with this syndrome include:
❏ Altered LOC (hypersomnolence or coma)
❏ Quadriparesis or quadreplegia (may have asymmetry)
❏ May have a "crossed paralysis," i.e., right face and left limbs or vice versa
❏ May have abnormal movements such as jerking, tremor, twitching, shivering. These movements may be misdiagnosed as seizure activity
❏ Oculomotor abnormalities; diplopia
 - These may include: <u>horizontal gaze palsy</u> (complete or unilateral), unilateral or bilateral internuclear ophthalmoplegia (INO), one and a half syndrome, skew deviation, gaze paretic nystagmus, bilateral ptosis, among others
❏ Pupillary abnormalities
 - May have pinpoint pupils
❏ Ataxia
❏ Bulbar symptoms (often bilateral)
 - These may include facial weakness, dysphagia, dysarthria, or dysphonia. Palatal myoclonus may be present
❏ Pseudobulbar affect

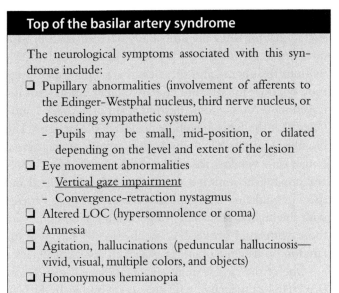

Top of the basilar artery syndrome

The neurological symptoms associated with this syndrome include:

- ❏ Pupillary abnormalities (involvement of afferents to the Edinger-Westphal nucleus, third nerve nucleus, or descending sympathetic system)
  - Pupils may be small, mid-position, or dilated depending on the level and extent of the lesion
- ❏ Eye movement abnormalities
  - <u>Vertical gaze impairment</u>
  - Convergence-retraction nystagmus
- ❏ Altered LOC (hypersomnolence or coma)
- ❏ Amnesia
- ❏ Agitation, hallucinations (peduncular hallucinosis—vivid, visual, multiple colors, and objects)
- ❏ Homonymous hemianopia

Some patients may have abnormal movements such as jerking, generalized tremor, twitching, or shivering which may be misinterpreted as seizure activity.

A patient with a brainstem stroke may become "locked-in" when there is paralysis of the limbs (quadriplegia) and face/mouth (cannot speak or move), AND they have retained cognition and alertness. Do not mistake this for coma. Locked-in patients are alert and able to communicate with their eyes, i.e., blinking and vertical eye movements. It results from damage to the pons affecting the corticospinal, corticobulbar, and corticopontine tracts with sparing of the higher centers.

Management of basilar artery occlusion

Patients with BAO were not included in the main tPA and EVT trials, so randomized data and treatment guidelines are currently lacking.

Observational (nonrandomized) studies have demonstrated that for BAO, the probability of recanalization with intravenous tPA or EVT is > 50% (compared with < 20% without treatment), and there can be a longer than usual time window for safe and effective intervention with intravenous tPA (extending beyond 4.5 h) or with EVT, provided that the brain imaging appearances look good. The biological rationale for why basilar occlusions can have a longer time window has been published.[1] However, a precise upper time limit has not yet been clearly defined and specific guideline recommendations are lacking. Patients with the highest probability of good clinical outcomes are those with mild stroke deficits, absence of extensive infarction on baseline brain imaging, and good collaterals.

One of the largest single-center prospective studies of BAO (184 consecutive patients) was reported by Strbian et al.[2] The majority (95%) were treated with intravenous tPA (plus heparin), 7% with mechanical thrombectomy, and 2% with intraarterial thrombolysis. Patients were treated up to 48-h post-onset (40% of patients were treated within 6-h post-onset and 60% were treated between 6 and 48 h post-onset). For patients who did not have extensive ischemic changes on baseline head CT (i.e. pc-ASPECTS score 8–10), recanalization was achieved in 73% of patients, and > 60% of those with recanalization achieved favorable clinical outcomes (modified Rankin score 0–3). The recanalization rates according to onset-to-treatment times were: 82% for patients treated within the first 6-h post-onset, 70% for those treated 6–12 h post-onset, and 75% for those treated 12–24 h post-onset.

The main factors associated with poor outcome were: older age, greater baseline clinical stroke severity (higher initial NIHSS score), lack of recanalization, and extensive ischemic changes on the baseline head CT.

In those without extensive baseline ischemic changes on CT, the time from stroke onset to treatment was not a significant predictor of clinical outcomes.

In the BASICS study[3] a prospective multicenter registry of patients with acute BAO, there were 27 patients who did not receive any treatment and 26/27 of them (96%) died within a month; the one survivor was left with severe disability and dependence. There were 409 patients who received treatment with either intravenous tPA or intraarterial therapy or combinations thereof. Overall, recanalization was achieved in 67% of the patients who received intravenous tPA and in 72% of patients who received intraarterial therapy. Earlier initiation of treatment was associated with a greater probability of surviving with a favorable functional outcome as compared with later treatment. In a subgroup of 114 patients who were treated within 9-h post-onset and were not already in a coma or a locked-in state or quadriplegic before treatment, 82% of the patients survived and 66% of the survivors had a favorable outcome (modified Rankin score 0–3 points). Conversely, for patients in this registry who had already developed severe deficits pretreatment (coma, quadriplegia, or locked-in state) and had their treatment initiated more than 9-h post-onset, none had a good outcome (all died or were left severely disabled).

A metaanalysis by Kumar et al.[4] of observational studies of reperfusion therapies for BAO pooled the results of 2056 patients from 45 studies published before August 2013. The overall recanalization rate was 75% (59% for intravenous thrombolysis and 77% for intraarterial/endovascular therapy). The recanalization rates were 81% for patients treated within 12-h post-onset and 73% for those treated > 12-h post-onset. Recanalization (compared to no recanalization) was associated with a twofold reduction in mortality and a 1.5-fold reduction in the rate of death or dependency.

The largest prospective cohort study of EVT for acute BAO published to date is the BASILAR study[5] – a nationwide registry involving 47 stroke centers in China that enrolled consecutive patients with acute symptomatic BAO (n=829) who could be treated within 24 of the estimated occlusion time. The results support the efficacy and safety of EVT for BAO. EVT achieved reperfusion in 81% of the patients. The proportion of EVT-treated patients who achieved a favorable functional recovery at 90 days (mRS score 0–3) was 32%. In the propensity score matching analysis, the proportion of patients achieving a favorable 90-day outcome (mRS score 0–3) was significantly higher among those who received EVT as compared with those who received standard medical therapy (28% vs. 10%; $p < .001$) and the 90-day mortality rate was lower (47 % vs. 70%; $p < .001$).

The BEST trial[6] randomized 131 patients in China to receive endovascular therapy plus standard medical therapy versus standard medical therapy alone within 8 hours of vertebrobasilar occlusion. The trial was terminated early due to high crossover rate (from control arm to interventional arm) and low recruitment, emphasizing the challenges of performing a randomized trial for BAO. In the main analysis (intention to treat), there was no evidence of difference in proportion of participants with mRS 0–3 at 90 days. However, in a secondary analysis, there was a higher rate of mRS 0–3 in those who actually received the intervention compared with those in the standard group (44% compared with 25%). Other randomized trials of EVT for BAO are currently underway.

Summary

In this chapter, we reviewed the diagnosis of acute basilar artery occlusion and the effect of recanalization treatments. Once considered an almost uniformly fatal type of stroke, with modern treatments BAO has become a potentially treatable condition for some patients. Randomized treatment trials are currently underway and may influence practice recommendations.

References and Further Reading

1. Lindsberg PJ, Pekkola J, Strbian D, et al. Time window for recanalization in basilar artery occlusion. Speculative synthesis. *Neurology.* 2015;85:1806–1815.

2. Strbian D, Sairanen T, Silvennoinen H, et al. Thrombolysis of basilar artery occlusion: impact of baseline ischemia and time. *Ann Neurol.* 2013;73:688–694.

3. Schonewille WJ, et al. Treatment and outcomes of acute basilar artery occlusion in the basilar artery international cooperation study (BASICS): a prospective registry study. *Lancet Neurol.* 2009;8:724–730.

4. Kumar G, Bavarsad Shahripour R, Alexandrov AV. Recanalization of acute basilar artery occlusion improves outcomes: a meta-analysis. *J Neurointerv Surg.* 2014;7(12):868–874.

5. Writing Group for the BASILAR Group. Assessment of Endovascular Treatment for Acute Basilar Artery Occlusion via a Nationwide Prospective Registry. *JAMA Neurol.* Published online February 20, 2020. https://doi/10.1001/jamaneurol.2020.0156.

6. Liu X, et al. Endovascular treatment versus standard medical treatment for vertebrobasilar artery occlusion (BEST): an open-label, randomised controlled trial. *Lancet Neurol.* 2020;19(12):115–122.

7. Mattle HP, Marcel A, Lindsberg PJ, et al. Basilar artery occlusion. *Lancet Neurol.* 2011;10:1002–1014.

CHAPTER 11

Acute stroke treatment: Acute blood pressure management and anticoagulation reversal

This chapter will provide you with an approach to blood pressure treatment in the acute stroke setting. We will review current best practice blood pressure recommendations for:
- ❏ Ischemic stroke patients ineligible for thrombolytic therapy.
- ❏ Ischemic stroke patients who are candidates for thrombolytic therapy, and blood pressure targets during and after thrombolytic administration, with a clinical vignette.
- ❏ Blood pressure management in the setting of acute intracerebral hemorrhage.

We will also review the management of anticoagulant-associated intracranial hemorrhage in the acute stroke setting.

Blood pressure (BP) control in the acute ischemic stroke setting requires a delicate balance. Very high blood pressure may increase cerebral edema or risk of hemorrhagic conversion. On the other hand, too rapid correction or precipitous falls in blood pressure can decrease cerebral perfusion pressure and worsen ischemia.

The Code Stroke Handbook © 2020 Elsevier Inc. All rights reserved.
https://doi.org/10.1016/B978-0-12-820522-8.00011-9

As per the current Canadian Stroke Best Practice Recommendations, patients who are not candidates for thrombolytic therapy should have their blood pressure lowered only if the systolic blood pressure is > 220 mmHg or if the diastolic blood pressure is > 120 mmHg.

For patients who are candidates for thrombolytic therapy, blood pressure should be < 185 mmHg systolic and < 110 mmHg diastolic. For the first 24 h after tPA administration, the blood pressure should be maintained below 180/105 mmHg to minimize the risk of intracerebral hemorrhage.

The choice of an intravenous antihypertensive agent should be based on current hypertension guidelines, which includes as first-line agents labetalol, hydralazine, or enalapril. Labetalol is typically used as the first-line agent given its quick and predictable mechanism to avoid precipitous drops. Caution should be used in patients with bradycardia, heart block, or asthma. A typical first dose is

Case presentation

A 55-year-old woman presents as a code stroke with a pure motor lacunar syndrome and is a candidate for tPA; however, her blood pressure is around 240/120 mmHg, and heart rate 85 bpm. The resident pushes 10-mg IV labetalol over 1 min with minimal effect. They repeat this 3 times (every 5 min), watching for bradycardia, and her blood pressure lowers to 200/110 mmHg and heart rate 77 bpm. A decision is made to start a labetalol infusion and after 15 min her blood pressure is 183/100 mmHg. TPA bolus is then administered and she is maintained on a labetalol infusion with a target blood pressure < 180/105 mmHg, with close observation of her heart rate to watch for bradycardia.

5–10 mg IV pushed over 1 min and repeated every 5 min as needed. After a few IV pushes, you should consider starting a labetalol infusion, especially to maintain blood pressure at target during the tPA infusion and afterward.

Intracerebral hemorrhage acute blood pressure management

In the setting of intracerebral hemorrhage, blood pressure should be closely monitored as high blood pressure has been associated with hematoma expansion and neurological deterioration. Recent clinical trials have tried to determine the optimal blood pressure target for patients presenting with intracerebral hemorrhage.

The **INTERACT 2 trial**[1] compared intensive versus standard reduction of blood pressure (with average systolic blood pressure reduction to 150 mmHg in the intensive group and 164 mmHg in the standard group). There was no overall difference in the rate of death or major disability between groups but there was a shift toward lower disability in the intensive BP treatment group.

The **ATACH 2 trial**[2] also compared intensive versus standard reduction, although blood pressure was reduced to a mean of 129 mmHg in the intensive group and 141 mmHg in the standard group. There was no difference in the rate of death or disability but higher rates of adverse renal events in those randomized to the intensive group.

Although the target blood pressure was the same in both trials, the ATACH 2 trial had a faster and more pronounced reduction of blood pressure. In the group that reached a mean blood pressure of 129 mmHg, there were more renal adverse events.

For patients presenting with acute intracerebral hemorrhage and elevated systolic BP between 150 and 220 mmHg, rapid BP lowering is recommended aiming for a target systolic BP of 140 mmHg, with intravenous antihypertensive medication and frequent BP monitoring.

For those with systolic BP > 220 mmHg, the optimal target is less clear and a target systolic BP of 140–160 mmHg is considered reasonable.

Management of anticoagulation-associated intracranial hemorrhage in the acute stroke setting

For patients presenting with acute intracranial hemorrhage, it is important to quickly determine whether or not the patient has a coagulopathy or is taking an anticoagulant medication (e.g. warfarin, heparin, apixaban, edoxaban, dabigatran, rivaroxaban; and find out the time of last dose taken). Get STAT INR, PTT, and platelet count.

Anticoagulant-associated intracranial hemorrhage is a life-threatening emergency. If the patient is taking warfarin with elevated INR, the recommended treatment is immediate administration of prothrombin complex concentrate, which is a rapidly-acting specific antidote for reversing warfarin (usually provided by the hospital Blood Bank; infused over 15–30 minutes, dosing depends on the INR level), in addition to a 10 mg dose of intravenous vitamin K, holding warfarin, and repeating INR at intervals to see if additional treatment is required. The antidote for heparin-associated hemorrhage is protamine sulfate. The specific antidote for dabigatran is idarucizumab, and for factor Xa inhibitors is andexanet alfa (FDA approved;

not currently available in Canada); both result in prompt reversal of serum anticoagulant levels. There are ongoing clinical trials evaluating these novel antidotes and in the interim prothrombin complex concentrate can be given for factor Xa inhibitor-associated hemorrhage. Tranexamic acid can also be considered in addition to the above reversal strategies for dabigatran or factor Xa inhibitors. For patients with severe thrombocytopenia, give a platelet transfusion. Protocols for reversal of anticoagulation may differ between hospitals and clinicians should refer to local hospital practices. Reversal agents should be administered as rapidly as possible after diagnosis of an anticoagulant-associated intracranial hemorrhage and in parallel with other management strategies including blood pressure reduction, critical care, or surgery.

Summary

Important best practice blood pressure recommended targets to remember are:

- ❏ < 185/110 mmHg—accepted cutoff for tPA eligibility.
- ❏ < 180/105 mmHg—for 24 h following tPA administration.
- ❏ Permissive hypertension (< 220/120 mmHg) is recommended for ischemic stroke patients not receiving acute intervention with tPA or EVT.
- ❏ In most cases of acute intracerebral hemorrhage, systolic BP should target between 140 and 160 mmHg.

Quickly identify if your patient has a coagulopathy or is taking an anticoagulant medication and administer specific reversal agents as rapidly as possible after diagnosis of an anticoagulant-associated intracranial hemorrhage.

References and Further Reading

1. Anderson CS, et al. Rapid blood-pressure lowering in patients with acute intracerebral hemorrhage. *N Engl J Med.* 2013;368(25):2355–2365.

2. Qureshi AI, et al. Intensive blood-pressure lowering in patients with acute cerebral hemorrhage. *N Engl J Med.* 2016;375(11):1033–1043.

3. Boulanger JM, et al. Canadian stroke best practice recommendations for acute stroke management: prehospital, emergency department, and acute inpatient stroke care, 6th edition, update 2018. *Int J Stroke.* 2018;13(9):949–984.

4. Butcher KS, et al. The intracerebral hemorrhage acutely decreasing arterial pressure trial. *Stroke.* 2013;44(3):620–626.

5. Hemphill JC, et al. Guidelines for the management of spontaneous intracerebral hemorrhage: a guideline for healthcare professional from the American Heart Association/American Stroke Association. *Stroke.* 2015;46(7):2032–2060.

6. Rabinstein A. Treatment of acute ischemic stroke. *Continuum.* 2017;23(1):62–81.

CHAPTER 12

Acute ischemic stroke treatment: Acute antiplatelet therapy

This chapter will provide a focused approach to antiplatelet therapy in the acute stroke setting for patients who are ineligible for tPA or EVT. We will review best practice recommendations regarding:
- ❏ The indications for single antiplatelet therapy
- ❏ The indications for dual antiplatelet therapy

1 Single antiplatelet therapy

Early treatment with aspirin (ASA) for patients with ischemic stroke who are not eligible for tPA or EVT has a small net benefit of reducing the risk of early recurrent stroke and death. According to a 2014 Cochrane review,[1] aspirin monotherapy given within 48 h of stroke onset resulted in a significant reduction in the odds of recurrent ischemic stroke, and death or functional dependence ($n=41,483$ patients). For every 1000 patients given ASA acutely, 9 deaths and 7 recurrent strokes will be prevented.

As per the Canadian Stroke Best Practice Recommendations, patients presenting with an ischemic stroke or TIA who are not eligible for acute intervention with tPA or EVT and are not on an antiplatelet agent at baseline should be loaded with ASA immediately (either orally if they have passed their swallowing assessment or rectally), unless there is an indication for dual antiplatelet therapy (DAPT) or anticoagulation.

The typical loading dose is ASA 160 mg orally, or 325 mg rectally. This should be followed by ASA 81 mg daily (unless there is an indication for DAPT or anticoagulation).

2 Dual antiplatelet therapy

A subset of patients with mild acute ischemic stroke (NIHSS 0–3) or high-risk TIA ($ABCD^2$ score ≥ 4) benefit from a short course of DAPT (ASA 81 mg + clopidogrel 75 mg daily) started as soon as possible after symptom onset, after head CT has excluded hemorrhage. This regimen for patients not receiving tPA or EVT is supported by the results of three trials (FASTER, CHANCE, and POINT) and metaanalysis.

The **CHANCE trial**,[2] in an exclusively Chinese population, provided evidence of benefit for a 3-week course of DAPT (started within 24 h of symptom onset) in patients with mild acute ischemic stroke (NIHSS 0–3) or high-risk TIA ($ABCD^2$ score ≥ 4), followed by single antiplatelet therapy thereafter. Fewer patients in the DAPT group experienced a new ischemic stroke within 90 days vs those who received ASA alone (8.2% vs 11.7%), a 30% relative reduction in stroke recurrence. There was no significant difference between groups in the rate of systemic or intracranial hemorrhage.

The **POINT trial**,[3] which enrolled the majority of patients from the United States, compared DAPT for 90 days vs ASA monotherapy in patients with an acute minor stroke (NIHSS 0–3) or high-risk TIA (ABCD^2 score ≥4) started within 12 h of symptom onset. Fewer patients in the DAPT group experienced a recurrent ischemic stroke within 90 days (4.6% vs 6.3%), with most of the stroke reduction occurring within the first week. Major hemorrhage (which includes systemic hemorrhage and symptomatic intracranial hemorrhage) occurred more frequently in the DAPT group compared with the single antiplatelet group (0.9% vs 0.4%) within 90 days; however, most of the bleeds occurred after 30 days. There was no significant difference between treatment groups in the rates of symptomatic ICH or hemorrhagic stroke. Importantly, although the eligibility criteria for enrollment in CHANCE and POINT were similar, the duration of DAPT was different (90 days for POINT and 21 days for CHANCE).

A **metaanalysis**[4] of the CHANCE, POINT, and FASTER trials involving over 10,000 patients established that the combination of aspirin and clopidogrel compared to single antiplatelet therapy after TIA or minor stroke reduced the risk of subsequent stroke by 20 in 1000 population (2% absolute benefit), predominantly within the first 10 days. The risk of major hemorrhage was small at 2 in 1000, and the risk accrued continuously over time. **For every 1000 patients treated with DAPT rather than ASA alone, 19 additional ischemic strokes would be prevented and two more major hemorrhages would occur.** For maximum net benefit, the recommended duration of DAPT is for the first 21 days after the index ischemic event.

In summary, patients with a minor nonhemorrhagic stroke (NIHSS 0–3) or high-risk TIA presenting within 24 h of symptom onset should be treated with aspirin 81 mg daily plus clopidogrel 75 mg daily, if no contraindication, for 21 days, followed thereafter by antiplatelet monotherapy (ASA or clopidogrel), unless there is an indication for anticoagulation, and provided they are not at high risk for bleeding.

Patients should be loaded with both ASA and clopidogrel. A typical loading dose for stroke treatment is 160 mg for ASA (followed by 81 mg daily), and 300 mg for clopidogrel (followed by 75 mg daily).

Patients with isolated sensory symptoms, isolated visual changes, isolated dizziness/vertigo, or a history of intracranial hemorrhage were excluded from these trials. In addition, patients with a modified Rankin scale score of > 2 (moderate disability at baseline) were also excluded. Dual antiplatelet therapy is not recommended for patients with moderate or large ischemic strokes, or patients at high risk for bleeding.

Case presentation

A 63-year-old woman was typing on the computer at work when she was suddenly unable to lift her left arm. She told her coworker who also noticed a facial droop and slurred speech. Her coworker immediately called 911. There were no accompanying neurological deficits. En route to the hospital, she recovered. She has a history of untreated sleep apnea and hypertension and takes an antihypertensive medication. No past medical history of bleeding or peptic ulcer.

Her blood pressure is 150/85 mmHg and heart rate is 98 bpm and regular. Her neurological examination is normal (NIHSS score = 0).

Noncontrast head CT scan and CTA of the head and neck arteries are unremarkable.

She was kept under observation in the ED and reassessed at intervals during the first 4.5 h of her symptoms onset, and she remained asymptomatic without any relapse or fluctuation of symptoms.

The diagnosis is a TIA, etiology not yet determined. She was assessed for tPA and was not a candidate given her spontaneous recovery and absence of clot on CTA. She passed her swallowing assessment and was loaded with aspirin 160 mg and clopidogrel 300 mg orally in the ED. She was felt to be in a low-risk category for bleeding. The rationale for DAPT and the benefits and risks were discussed with her. She was given instructions to take aspirin 81 mg daily and clopidogrel 75 mg daily for 21 days and then to stop clopidogrel and continue aspirin 81-mg daily indefinitely for secondary stroke prevention. A full etiological stroke workup was planned, including ECG monitoring and echocardiography to investigate for paroxysmal atrial fibrillation or other cardiac source of embolism.

What if the patient has an ischemic stroke on antiplatelet monotherapy and is not a candidate for DAPT?

At the present time, there is insufficient evidence to guide management in this case. Clinicians often choose to switch to a different antiplatelet (e.g., switching from aspirin to clopidogrel monotherapy). A full review of potential causes of recurrent stroke should be pursued, and all vascular risk factors should be optimized and aggressively managed.

Summary

We reviewed the indication, dose, and route of administration of single antiplatelet therapy for patients not candidates for acute reperfusion therapy with tPA or EVT.

Indications for DAPT (for 21 days) for patients presenting with a TIA or mild ischemic stroke and not receiving tPA or EVT include an NIHSS score 0–3 or high risk TIA. Consideration of stroke mimics is important for this patient population to avoid overtreatment.

References and Further Reading

1. Sandercock PA, Counsell C, Tseng MC, Cecconi E. Oral antiplatelet therapy for acute ischaemic stroke. *Cochrane Database Syst Rev.* 2014;3:CD000029.
2. Wang Y, et al. Clopidogrel with aspirin in acute minor stroke or transient ischemic attack. *N Engl J Med.* 2013;369(1):11–19.
3. Johnston SC, et al. Clopidogrel and aspirin in acute ischemic stroke and high-risk TIA. *N Engl J Med.* 2018;379(3):215–225.
4. Hao Q, et al. Clopidogrel plus aspirin versus aspirin alone for acute minor ischaemic stroke or high risk transient ischaemic attack: systematic review and meta-analysis. *BMJ.* 2018;363:k5108.
5. Boulanger JM, et al. Canadian stroke best practice recommendations for acute stroke management: prehospital, emergency department, and acute inpatient stroke care, 6th edition, update 2018. *Int J Stroke.* 2018;13(9):949–984.
6. Johnston SC, Elm JJ, Easton JD, et al. On behalf of the POINT and Neurological Emergencies Treatment Trials Network Investigators. Time course for benefit and risk of clopidogrel and aspirin after acute transient ischemic attack and minor ischemic stroke: a secondary analysis from the POINT randomized trial. *Circulation.* 2019;140(8):658–664.
7. Kennedy J, Hill MD, Ryckborst KJ, et al. Fast assessment of stroke and transient ischaemic attack to prevent early recurrence (FASTER): a randomised controlled pilot trial. *Lancet Neurol.* 2007;6(11):961–969.

Index

Note: Page numbers followed by *f* indicate figures, *t* indicate tables, and *b* indicate boxes.

9780128205228